Raw Material

Raw Material

PRODUCING PATHOLOGY IN VICTORIAN CULTURE

❧ *Erin O'Connor*

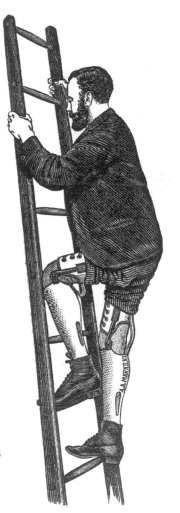

DUKE UNIVERSITY PRESS

Durham & London, 2000

Designed by Rebecca M. Giménez
Typeset in Caslon by Keystone Typesetting, Inc.
Frontispiece: "Climbing the Evolutionary Ladder"
From A. A. Marks, *Treatise on Marks' Patent
Artificial Limbs with Rubber Hands and Feet* (1888).
Library of Congress Cataloging-in-Publication
Data appear on the last printed page of this book.
An earlier version of chapter 3 was published
in *Comparative Studies in Society and History*,
and is reprinted with the permission of
Cambridge University Press.

BODY, COMMODITY, TEXT

Studies of Objectifying Practice

A series edited by Arjun Appadurai,

Jean Comaroff, and Judith Farquhar

❧ CONTENTS

❧ FIGURES

❧ ACKNOWLEDGMENTS

Writing this book has alternately been a labor of love and a lesson in living. Over the six years of its making, *Raw Material* has been both solace and incubus, pleasure and burden by turns. It has had to be coaxed, tickled, wrestled, fought, and laughed into being, and its difficulties and its joys have over time resolved themselves into a private joke; like Mr. Venus, eternally anxious about the respectability of his trade in bones, I have found myself countless times grumbling his immortal lines at my recalcitrant manuscript: "Don't sauce *me*, in the wicious pride of your youth; don't hit *me* because you see I'm down. You've no idea how small you'd come out if I had the articulating of you." Well, now we know: I hope it's satisfied. Many people and institutions have had a hand in the articulating of *Raw Material,* and I am glad to be able to thank them here.

I owe special thanks to my teachers at the University of Michigan, who saw this project through its earliest incarnations as coursework and dissertation. For introducing me to interdisciplinary work, and for managing somehow to provide excellent advice, criticism, and guidance while still giving me the freedom to follow the unpredictable path of my ideas, I thank John Kucich, Martin Pernick, Adela Pinch, Martha Vicinus, and Athena Vrettos. Always to me a living example—to invert Dickens's words—of How To Do It, they continue to inspire and teach me. My colleagues at the University of Pennsylvania have been similarly generous with their time, creativity, and support. Nina Auerbach's uncanny critical imagination, David Delaura's finely tuned sensitivity to detail, and Elaine Freedgood's like mind all left their special marks on the manuscript at crucial moments in its evolution from dissertation to book; without them it would be raw material indeed. It has been my great good luck to have had such excellent intellectual company, both at Penn and at Michigan. My secret life as an other Victorian has been filled with a type of sympathy George Eliot would have trembled—pleasurably, I hope—to see; truly it has had the kind of beauty that is thrown into relief by poor dress.

So many other smart and interested readers have helped this book along over the years: Jonathan Freedman, Sander Gilman, Jill Matus, Dianne Sadoff, and an anonymous reader for Duke University Press all read the whole and made astute and helpful suggestions. Seth Koven and Thomas Laqueur read earlier versions of the amputation chapter and made careful, clarifying comments. Laurel Erickson, Jean Leverich, and Jani Scandura patiently sorted through drafts, often at odd hours and on short notice. Christine Cooper has ever been a faithful reader, creative listener, tireless interlocutor, fellow yogaholic, and consummate friend. Robyn Scherr and Dana Barton, who live and work in the real world, committed the remarkable act of reading this work for pleasure, and so reminded me of my reason for writing in the first place. Maurice Black brought to the book an almost visionary intelligence and a finely focused editorial eye. Much of my thinking about cultural theory was honed during our conversations, and much of my language was tightened at his suggestion. His care with details, and his challenging questions, have made this a far better book than it otherwise would have been. Ken Wissoker, Katie Courtland, Melinda Conner, Rebecca M. Giménez, and Patricia Mickelberry at Duke proved to me that university presses can be both human and humane; they will never know how much I appreciate their patience, openness, encouragement, and all-around reasonableness.

As a heavy and not always well-behaved user of libraries, I owe particular thanks to the archives I have exploited and the librarians who have tolerated my often intractable borrowing habits. Thanks to the Harlan Hatcher Graduate Library and the Taubman Medical Library at Michigan for forgiving fees, bending borrowing policies, and extending my interlibrary loans for years at a time. Thanks to Van Pelt Library at Penn for same, especially to John Pollack of Special Collections for letting me photograph disintegrating books, and to the University Photographic Services for making faded and blurry images beautifully clear. Thanks to the College of Physicians of Philadelphia, especially Chris Stanwood and Gretchen Worden, for graciously permitting me to photograph both disintegrating books and disintegrating photographs; to Carolyn Davis, of Special Collections at Syracuse; to the Barnum Museum; to Ricky Jay; and to the Circus World Museum for permission to reprint their images of monsters. Shanyn Fiske labored heroically checking quotes, chasing down sources, procuring permissions, and prodding photographers.

My thanks also to the University of Michigan for generous financial support during the dissertation phase. A Mellon Candidacy Fellowship, a Rackham Predoctoral Fellowship, and a Rackham One-Term Fellowship all secured me precious untrammeled writing time.

My deepest thanks go to my family, whose love, friendship, faith, and chronic irreverence planted the germ of this book in me years ago. Some of my earliest memories are of ogling the pictures in medical books while my mother studied for her boards; of smelling formaldehyde on my anatomist father when he picked me up from day care on dissection day; of the quirky anatomical decor of our scientific house (Bones, warious. Skulls, warious. Bottled preparations, warious. That's the general panoramic view); and of my own announcement at around age six that I would be a writer when I grew up. For understanding my need to read and write, for teaching me to combine labor with creation, and for raising me in the modern equivalent of Mr. Venus's shop, I thank you from the bottom of my freeze-dried heart. This book is for you.

In his 1843 critique of industrialism, *Past and Present,* Thomas Carlyle describes the Condition of England as one of terminal illness: "England is full of wealth, of multifarious produce, supply for human want in every kind; yet England is dying of inanition" (7). Imagining England as a spent and exhausted body, Carlyle suggests that the trouble with the nation is consumption. Like the tubercular, or consumptive, body, which was commonly believed to suffer from a "perverted or imperfect nutrition" (Greenhow 19), the body of England is dying not from lack of nourishment (in this case, goods), but rather from a systematic failure to distribute those goods in an efficient or effective way: "What is the use of your spun shirts?" Carlyle asks. "They hang there by the million unsaleable; and here, by the million, are diligent bare backs that can get no hold of them. Shirts are useful for covering human backs; unless otherwise, an unbearable mockery otherwise" (27). In Carlyle's logic, capitalism describes a cultural pathology in which a constitutional inability to assimilate wealth produces an increasingly enfeebled and diminished social body; unable to make use of its own material resources, able to produce but not to consume, commercialized England is literally wasting away.[1]

Carlyle's image of a consumptive England was more than merely metaphorical: nineteenth-century England really was dying of consumption. Where Carlyle and others diagnosed a social body incapable of surviving the advent of consumer culture, doctors noted that consumptive disease was itself reaching epidemic proportions (between 1838 and 1839, for instance, consumption—also known as pthisis and, increasingly, as tuberculosis—caused more than sixty thousand deaths in England and Wales alone). The nineteenth century saw both the consolidation of the mass market and the massive spread of consumptive disease, which followed the patterns of urbanization with deadly accuracy.[2] The century's number one killer, consumption spread fastest in cities and infected disproportionate numbers of the poor. As such, it operated as a kind of pathological index of demographic shift, a sickening sign of England's transformation from a primarily rural, agrarian nation to the world's first and foremost manufacturing economy. Carlyle's image of a state consumed by mass production thus found its material counterpart in actual patterns of tubercular spread, which mapped a nation of consumptive producers: "If one roams the streets a little in the early morning, when the multitudes are on their way to their work," Engels writes in *The Condition of the Working Class in England* (1845), "one is amazed at the number of persons who look wholly or half-consumptive." London was, naturally, the capital of this sickly culture of consumption. "Even in Manchester," Engels continues, "the people have not the same appearance: these pale, lank, narrow-chested, hollow-eyed ghosts, whom one passes at every step, these languid, flabby faces, incapable of the slightest energetic expression, I have seen in such startling numbers only in London" (109). For Engels, consumption doesn't just affect the working classes, it defines them: the picture of poor health, they are the spitting (and coughing) images of Carlyle's wasted, wasting social body.

Infecting millions of people and informing political critique, consumption was one of the nineteenth century's enduring cultural and medical problems. Absolutely symptomatic of industrial existence, consumption described what doctors, in a somewhat different context, called a "pthisical habitus," a symbolic economy in which the pathological conditions of consumption and the Condition of England continually indicated each other.[3] Bringing up complementary images of poorly paid labor and hard, labored breathing; of airless rooms and ill-ventilated chests; consumption spoke of a decomposition that was taking place on both social and cellular levels, a decomposition that drew the diseased body into such close contact with social disorder that it became difficult to tell them apart: if stuffy interiors were felt to be a principal cause of consumption, breath that reeked of a "newly-plastered room" was a dead giveaway of advancing pulmonary disease (Cotton 118). Consumption raised all sorts of hectic, hellish associations, simultaneously imaging dark, damp courts and rank, rotting sores; noxious vapors and obnoxious breath; stagnant pools of sewage and pints of spewed blood; bad drainage and draining pus; choked privies and endless plugs of putrid sputum, the sticky seals of respiratory distress. More than anything else, the products of consumptive coughing circulated the ugly truth about the system. Alternately clear, white, yellow, green, or gray, they were streaked with black matter and shot through with clots. Hawks from strangled lungs were ubiquitous, festering on floors and mucking up streets; sitting in chamber pots and saturating sheets; smeared on handkerchiefs, sleeves, and the backs of hands; crusting into dust and eventually entering other lungs on clouds of vitiated air. The hallmarks of universal infection, widespread destitution, and awful, early death, they were the terribly expressive signs of an increasingly invalid world. At once a killer figure for an emergent mass culture and a material condition *of* that culture, consumption had a phenomenal career during the nineteenth century.

The word *consumption* articulates a convergence that is everywhere apparent in nineteenth-century thinking: where social critics diagnosed England as a diseased and dying body, disease itself provided a gross anatomy of the social system. This book concerns itself with the complexities of this formation, analyzing the inextricable entangling of ideas about capitalism and corporeality in Victorian discourses of disease. It studies the poetics of pathology during the nineteenth century, examining how the material patterns of disease became the basis for a highly metaphorical exploration of the human condition.[4] Drawing on medicine, literature, political economy, sociology, anthropology, and popular advertising, this work explores the industrial logic of disease in Victorian culture, the dynamic coupling of pathology and production in Victorian thinking about cultural processes in general, and about disease in particular. It centers on the epistemological continuity between the disorderly materiality of unhealthy bodies and the radically altered social order of an increasingly materialist culture, examining how the forms and figures of urban industrial disorder filtered through the language surrounding actual disease. Paying particular attention to how the exigencies of the material body were explained by—and as— problems of material culture, this book traces how the language of disease continually aligns pathological processes with social forces. In so doing, it seeks to show how anxieties about cultural shift informed and sometimes merged with models of disease, and to situate those models within a set of broad concerns regarding the status of the human body under capitalism.[5]

The conceptual conjunction between pathology and production in Victorian thinking is perhaps most succinctly expressed in what Ruskin refers to in *Unto This Last* (1860) as "illth," a term that combines illness and wealth into a single category of biosocial detritus (105). Suggesting that "ill" effects are built into progress, that economic development necessarily involves some form of physical decay, *illth* both demarcates an imaginative fusion of body and money and designates that fusion as inherently pathological: illth implies a physicality whose unhealthy economic relations render it always already unwell. As Catherine Gallagher has pointed out, the viability of money in Ruskin's logic depends on the well-being, or "valor" ("The Bio-Economics of *Our Mutual Friend*" 99), of its possessor; a dead man cannot technically be rich because he cannot spend, and a living man who does not know how to use his resources cannot properly be said to be alive, precisely because his money is not circulating.[6] Such men are "inherently and eternally incapable of wealth"—they are "in reality no more wealthy than the locks of their own strong boxes"—and this incapacity renders them incapable of life (104). At best, they are merely "animated conditions of delay" (105); at worst, they are "as pools of dead water, and eddies in a stream (which, so long as the stream flows, are useless, or serve only to drown people)" (104). Imagining a perfect correspondence between civic responsibility and bodily health, illth describes an economy in which those who are wasteful will themselves waste away. We might take illth as a metaphor for Victorian models of pathology, which not only overlap with ideas about production at various points but are also embedded in a wider investigation of the relationship between physical and economic well-being. Where Victorian political economy orga-

nized social critique around questions of bodily health, medical literature developed a political economy of pathology, a rhetoric of human
physiology in which disease figures, paradoxically, as a profoundly productive degenerative force. Illth imagines a deeply elemental relationship between wasting and disease, casting death as an objectification
of the body—the man who is "inherently and eternally incapable of
wealth" is not a dead man but a pool of dead water; *he* doesn't drown
people, but the thing he has been reduced to *does*. In illth, the body
wastes into waste itself.

This imaginary fusion of trash and flesh must be understood in the
context of nineteenth-century debates about the impact of industry on
public health, and, more specifically, about the vexed and uncertain
relationship between the human body and the raw materials of manufacture. The rise of the factory system and the attendant growth of
cities during the nineteenth century caused a national health crisis,
subjecting people in ever greater numbers to the killing effects of economic growth.[7] Works such as James Phillips Kay's *Moral and Physical
Condition of the Working Classes Employed in the Cotton Manufacture in
Manchester* (1832), Edwin Chadwick's *Report on the Sanitary Condition
of the Labouring Population of Great Britain* (1842), and Friedrich Engels's *Condition of the Working Class in England* (1845) offer elaborate
accounts of how the living conditions in urban slums contributed to the
spread of infectious diseases such as typhoid, smallpox, cholera, influenza, and scarlet fever, as well as how extreme poverty and overwork
fostered a range of constitutional disorders. Known colloquially as
"fever nests," the slums' lack of ventilation and fresh water, inadequate
sanitation, and severe overcrowding encouraged epidemics and exacer-
bated disorders arising from malnutrition such as rickets, scurvy, and
anemia. Disease was the most visible index of the decisive power of
urban squalor to squelch human life. Despite important medical advancements such as improved diagnostic and therapeutic techniques,
anesthesia, and antisepsis, and despite an increasing number of public
health measures devoted to providing better sanitation and purer water,
cities took an unbelievable toll on health.[8] Life expectancy in the cities
was exceptionally low, especially among the poor. Most people never
made it past middle age, and between industrial accidents and grinding
poverty, workers were lucky to see thirty.[9] Infant mortality was corre-

spondingly high: every year, more than 100,000 English babies died
before reaching their first birthday (Wohl 11). Contagion and prevention were poorly understood, allowing epidemics to sweep through
slums and suburbs with devastating regularity: in 1847–48, influenza
killed 50,000 people in London alone; scarlet fever killed 34,000 people
in 1863, and more than 26,000 in 1874; almost 42,000 people died of
smallpox between 1837 and 1840 (Wohl 128–33). Typhus was mild by
comparison: in 1869, when it was first differentiated from typhoid, it
killed 4,281 in England and Wales (Wohl 125).

In addition to creating urban conditions that facilitated the spread of
extant diseases, industrialism generated a whole series of new ones. The
publication of Charles Turner Thackrah's revised and expanded *Effects
of Arts, Trades, and Professions on Health and Longevity* in 1832, and the
subsequent proliferation of parliamentary reports on the working conditions of trades, marked the advent of a highly technical concern with
the relationship between work and the body that was to last well into the
twentieth century.[10] Indeed, Victorian writing about "industrial diseases," pathologies that were the direct results of working conditions,
forms a distinct genre of social critique. Thackrah's treatise, which
divides diseases by trade—despite considerable overlap among occupations—and devotes as much attention to the nature of the work that
caused disease as it does to diseases themselves, set the standard for
subsequent treatments of the subject. Over the course of the century,
these reports established a normative model for thinking about the link
between illness and work. In identifying the ailments common to specific occupations—indeed, by identifying certain occupations with specific ailments—they framed disease as something that was itself custom-
made, the product of a highly specialized interaction between body and
machine, human flesh and raw material. This association was encoded
in the names given to the more idiosyncratic industrial pathologies—
"grinder's asthma," "potter's rot," and "brassfounder's ague" all express a
proprietary attitude toward disease, a sense that certain pathological
formations "belong" to certain work operations, that they are as much a
product of labor as commodities themselves. In representing disease as
something that is made by work—even at times representing work as a
pathogenic operation in itself—Victorian writing about industrial dis-

ease elides body and commodity by positioning the diseased body of the worker as the outcome of his labor. Whether conservative (as in Chadwick's laissez-faire politics) or radical (as in Engels's socialism), this literature consistently forwards the notion that what the factory system really mass-produces is pathology itself.

If critiques of the factory system situate disease as the end product of labor, they also represent the worker's body as a quantity of raw material that is subjected to a laborious, painful, and ultimately useless course of manufacture. According to these studies, industrial disease remade the worker's body in the image of his trade. Jobs involving repetitive mechanical movements, for instance, tended to cause unusual orthopedic problems, generating joint deformities, permanent flexures, and even paralyses that embodied the adaptive subordination of body parts to specific tools and machines. Engels describes a condition called "hind-leg," particular to lathe workers who had "from perpetually filing at the lathe, crooked backs and one leg crooked . . . so that the two legs have the form of a K" (210), while an 1869 *Lancet* article anatomizes a condition called "hephaestic hemiplegia," or "hammer palsy," in which prolonged use of a seven-pound hammer caused gradual paralysis over the entire right sides of carpenters' bodies (quoted in Arlidge 554). In these disorders, workers' bodies were overtaken by the work performance; physical disability marked the worker's complete appropriation by the activity and apparatus of labor. J. T. Arlidge's exhaustive *Hygiene Diseases and Mortality of Occupations* (1892) contains numerous such examples. "Silk twisting," for instance, in which boys ran back and forth while holding a heavy skein of thread at arm's length, caused a corresponding "twisting of the trunk to that side"; the resulting spinal curvature and knee deformities represented a pathological embedding of the work activity in the body's structure, a debilitating confusion of act and object, cause and effect: the twister finally became so twisted that he could no longer perform the act of twisting (557). Similarly, button makers suffered from "choreitic movements of the hands and fingers . . . due to erethism of the nerve centres of the brain from perpetually dealing with minute objects in a monotonous fashion" (555); even at rest their hands habitually fluttered through the routinized motions of their work (as such, button makers tragically realized the productive ideal of having certain skills at one's fingertips). In these examples, labor reforms the body in its own image, twisting, bending, and stiffening it into postures that are at once perfectly adaptive and acutely pathological. Indeed, debilitated workers frequently reported that they preferred the very cramped, hunched-over positions that helped to produce their complaints. Engels notes that metal grinders suffering from respiratory failure compensated for their shortness of breath by obstructing their own freedom of movement. In an all-too-literal enactment of labored breathing, "they habitually raise the shoulders to relieve the permanent and increasing want of breath; they bend forward, and seem, in general, to feel most comfortable in the crouching position in which they work" (211–12).

Where some workers were so thoroughly worked over that they came to embody the specific motions of their own labor, others were chemically altered by their own raw materials. Jobs requiring workers to handle toxic substances such as lead, arsenic, and phosphorus; to breathe noxious fumes from naphtha, turpentine, and petroleum; or to inhale the thick dust from textile manufacture, bone and metal grinding, and coal mining, led to systemic problems such as slow poisoning, chronic respiratory failure, and progressive nerve damage. These disorders involved a kind of corporeal amalgamation, a merging of workers' bodies with the raw materials of their trades. This pathological combination of flesh and raw material was dramatically contained in the phlegmatic formations of workers suffering from industrial asthma. Metal grinders, for instance, coughed up balls of phlegm composed of mucus and metallic dust (Engels 212), while colliers produced spittle blackened by coal. In "grinder's asthma" and "black spit" the body's refuse revealed the raw materials of its trade: the grinder's expectorations marked his efforts to expel the needlelike metal fragments piercing his bronchial tubes, while the miner's charred saliva registered the fact that his lungs were clogged with coal. Industrial diseases thus incorporated an entire problematic of materiality, emerging precisely at the point where the raw materials of industry—flecks of glass, metal splinters, textile dust, toxic fumes—entered the human body, embedding themselves in the tissues of the lungs, seeping through the skin into the bloodstream, collecting in the bones and liver and brain.

This problematic relation, in which manufacture altered bodily composition, took a variety of forms: industrial disease manifested itself as an adaptation of parts, as when the skeleton deformed itself to fit a machine; as a mixing of human and industrial waste, as in metallic mucus or lumps of phlegmatic coal; and, most dramatically, as a chemical reaction between flesh and raw material. Copper poisoning, for instance, converted the worker into a kind of anatomical alloy; smelters absorbed so much metal that they acquired its chemical properties. They tasted like copper—coughing up dust leaves a "metallic, coppery taste" (Arlidge 442) in workers' mouths—and they even oxidized: as copper molecules fused with oxygen in the body's tissues, the hair, gums, urine and stools all took on a greenish tint (442–44). Likewise, matchmakers suffering from phosphorus poisoning became phosphorescent. As the phosphorus penetrated into the jaw and spread to the surrounding tissues of the head and neck, workers laboring under matchmaker's necrosis began to glow; indeed, with their luminously decomposing heads atop comparatively inert bodies, matchmakers with "phossy jaw" were living lucifer matches in their own right.[11] Industrial diseases thus incorporated a process in which the compounding of tissue and toxin was so thorough that they could no longer be told apart.

The imaginative significance of industrial diseases—as signs of inhumane working conditions, and, more broadly, as evidence of how industrial capitalism reconfigures the body—can be seen in Elizabeth Gaskell's novel *North and South* (1855), wherein a character named Bessy Higgins dies of respiratory failure after working in an unventilated Manchester cotton mill. Troubled by a chronic cough and increasingly unable to breathe, she attributes her asthmatic condition to "fluff. . . . Little bits, as fly off fro' the cotton, when they're carding it, and fill the air till it looks all fine white dust. They say it winds round the lungs, and tightens them up. Anyhow, there's many a one as works in a carding-room, that falls into a waste, coughing and spitting blood, because they're just poisoned by the fluff" (146). Although Bessy's image of the strangulating action of fluff is highly impressionistic, not to mention anatomically impossible (dust breathed into the lungs could never wrap itself around them), the basic impulse behind her description is technically correct: industrial diseases embody a process by which the material body and the raw materials of industry become hopelessly intertwined.

It is in this context that we can begin to understand the figurative connection between disease and industry in Victorian medical literature. The material patterns of industrial pathology found a metaphorical counterpart in medical models of disease, which mapped productive language onto pathological process as a means of investigating the meaning of corporeality in machine culture. The chapters that follow study various dimensions of this broad dynamic. Organized by disease, *Raw Material* is made up of four case studies that work together to show how the specific manifestations of individual diseases became the means of investigating the effect of "progress" on personhood. Chapter 1 focuses on the deadly modern plague, Asiatic cholera. An Eastern disease that ravaged England on four separate occasions between 1831 and 1865, cholera materialized anxieties about cultural contamination. Brought over from India on ships and then circulated through the streets of English cities, it provided a figure for the threatening fluidity of cultural and bodily boundaries in an imperialist world economy. By looking at how choleric pathology came to be symptomatic of the wider degenerative patterns of machine culture, this chapter lays the groundwork for later ones by raising questions about the relationship between materiality and metaphor in Victorian thought. Chapter 2 shows how a conceptual antipathy between femininity and the factory system modulated the social construction of breast cancer. Describing malignant masses as mass productions, the discourse of breast cancer drew on the vocabulary of machine culture to develop an "objective" approach to a heartbreakingly invasive and all-but-incurable disease. The third chapter extends this investigation of how mechanization affected models of selfhood. Assessing the impact of dismemberment and prosthesis on notions of working-class masculinity, it shows how, in merging male bodies with machines, prosthetics reconstituted injured soldiers and industrial workers through a utilitarian model of gender: by restoring physical mobility, artificial limbs suggested that all a man needed to be truly himself was a working body. Chapter 4 anatomizes the symbolic importance of deformity for Victorian culture, analyzing how the freak show opened up a space for considering objectification as a strategy of selfhood—one that was uniquely suited to the demands of a culture increasingly organized around the production and consumption of goods.

Conceptually, the book is divided into two halves. The first half concentrates on nightmares of physical dissolution. Asiatic cholera and cancer were violent and invasive; their onset was frequently sudden, and their progress often excruciatingly painful. Victims of these diseases absolutely disintegrated, their bodies dissolving so thoroughly into dead matter that their corpses bore little resemblance to the people that had once animated them. Stinking and stiff with rigor, they showed how desperately ill equipped the human body was to meet the specific environmental challenges of modern life. Moreover, Asiatic cholera and breast cancer not only killed their victims but also metaphorically obliterated their status as people. Asiatic cholera staged a traumatic transformation of white, working-class flesh into worthless black stuff—in medicine and popular journalism the dark, dehydrated corpse of the cholera victim is likened to tar, coal, pitch, and even feces. Similarly, the wasting of the body in breast cancer took shape as a commodification of the flesh. Tumors were treated as scenes of mass production, as factories that transformed female tissue into rotten imitations of market items—bad eggs, rank cheese, squishy fruit. By representing disease as a course of material transformation, the language surrounding these conditions embodied a crisis of modernization, imaging the impasse between what bodies are and what the world was becoming by symbolically dissolving flesh into the nasty smells, rank fluids, and filthy scraps of the slum. Portraying dying bodies as bodies blurring into the gross residuum of city space, they provided a way of talking about how the self was dying, a way of symbolically trashing the notion that people are essentially different from—and more valuable than—more mundane materials. The second half of the book shifts to an examination of how pathology could foster dreams of symbolic and social resolution, analyzing how the loss of bodily boundaries that was so threatening in cholera and cancer could become constitutive of new models of identity. Where the darkened and dehydrated bodies of cholera victims symbolically devolved into piles of industrial dirt and women with breast cancer degenerated into rhetorical analogues of inner cities, prosthetics and the freak show effected a therapeutic recuperation of the radically disfigured body through a tactical commodification. In amputation and deformity, disfiguring injuries and birth defects made it possible to rework the contours of industrial identity. Prosthetics and monsters rebuilt the self by taking bodily anomaly as the condition of a new personal integrity. Framing amputees as whole men with artificial limbs and marketing monsters as "living curiosities" worked paradoxically to secure their humanity by objectifying them.

In conceiving of pathology as a course of material transformation, a process through which the sentient, thinking subject is reduced and reconstituted, compounded—sometimes violently, sometimes profitably—into new metaphorical and material compositions, the logics of cholera, cancer, prosthesis, and monstrosity raise a series of questions about the place of the body in forming human identity. The middle chapters thus pair to form a detailed examination of how gender fits into logics of bodily mutilation and repair. Where analogies between the degenerative course of a woman's disease and the urban decay of the industrial city enabled doctors to face—and finally perfect—mastectomy, writing about dismemberment treats technology as an antidote to the pathology of amputation, asserting that prosthetic machines can re-create the essence of a man. Each discourse posits an elemental affinity between the material body and material culture, suggesting that their basic processes and properties reflect each other. And yet, in refracting that affinity through gender, they arrive at profoundly different conclusions about what such an alignment means. In the one, it becomes a way of making a woman's disease ungendered, and therefore manageable; in the other, it manages the disturbing neuropathy of limb loss by framing it as a far more comprehensible problem of embattled manhood.

Likewise, both Asiatic cholera and monstrosity display dramatically different attitudes about racial stability. Cholera kills by dehydration: vomiting and diarrhea drained victims of so much fluid that within days or even hours they were reduced to darkened, dried-up fragments of their former selves. This darkening and drying in turn condensed widespread anxieties about whether industrial development was occurring at the expense of the English "race." In the absence of satisfying explanations for epidemic spread, doctors and popular writers alike made cholera into a parable of substantial speciation, a dark fable of national decline in which the blackening of the victim's body blots out Englishness itself. By contrast, the bodies of human monsters became a means of promoting a new, improved image of the modern individual. Where Asiatic cholera framed a horror story of national annihilation, the freak show sold spectacular physical degeneration as the condition of self-realization. In the one, pathology makes visible the sheer fragility of white, Western identity, its utter vulnerability to the social conditions of modernity. In the other, a carnivalesque iconography of an indestructible, industrial-strength self emerges, one whose amazing flaws work ironically to signify its social worth. The first and last chapters thus provide complementary accounts of working-class identity: monstrosity figures as a kind of fun-house reflection of cholera, a curious celebration of the very patterns of objectification that haunt the rhetoric of epidemic spread.

Taken together, these diseases have much to tell us about not only how Victorians thought the body, but also how the body helped Victorians think; indeed, they might be said to constitute an elaborate meditation on the impact of industrialism on selfhood. Nineteenth-century figurations of cholera, cancer, amputation, and deformity situate the body as a liminal material space between self and world, at once the scene of self-confirmation and the volatile, vulnerable stuff of self-annihilation. As such, they became occasions for expressing fears about what modernization was doing to bodies and the selves inside them, as well as fantasies about what sort of body was best suited for survival in an unstable industrial world. Pathology thus drove a massive act of cultural imagining: if it made visible the horrible vulnerability of flesh to the exigencies of modern life, its utter inability to maintain its essential integrity in the face of industrial culture, it also supplied a powerful means of metaphorically reforming the self. Damaged, diseased flesh was more than just a symptom of social destruction; it was also the raw material of a new kind of personhood, one that made the ailing individual into a kind of gross national product, a working endorsement for the very culture that injured and exploited him. Moving from degeneration to regeneration, *Raw Material* thus charts how Victorians used disease to stage the symbolic dissolution of the British self and to reformulate that self from the very materials that had threatened to destroy it.

It is by now a truism that the Victorians saw the human body as a source of ultimate truth, a way of knowing the world. In an era of optimistic positivism, the body was felt to naturalize social hierarchies based on race, gender, and class, and so to provide biological justification for the rigid social ordering built into capitalism and global expansion. Emergent scientific discourses of the body shared certain basic assumptions about the relationship of body to self, and of self to world; in works as diverse as Acton and Greg's studies of prostitution, Chadwick's sanitary reports, Galton's eugenics, Lombroso's criminal anthropology, Maudsley's psychology, Mayhew's urban profiles, and Spencer's sociology we see the same sorts of ideas at work again and again: that social roles were scripted by biology; that sexual, racial, and class differences were written into one's features, tissues, and cells; that one's place in the world was largely inherited, preordained by natural law. Above all, Victorian logics of embodiment sought certainty; they found out the way of the world by tautology, ordering culture by ordering the body, ordering the body by discovering in it the germ of social structure. Together, these logics projected a body so hermeneutically stable that even its more erratic incarnations could only ever speak the truth of their nature. So it was that Lombroso could detect criminal tendencies in cranial structure, that Pauline Tarnowsky could diagnose fallen women in flawed earlobes, and that Cuvier could dissect the bestial truth of black female sexuality in the distinctive labia and buttocks of the female Hottentot.[12] The murderer's skull and teeth, the prostitute's ear, and the Hottentot's genitalia—not to mention the more mundane markers of skin color, sex, and personal appearance—all told a story of identity thoroughly embodied, of selves so elaborately materialized that one's moral, mental, and emotional fibers could be read in the telling characters of flesh and bone. The biological determinism of so much Victorian thinking was thus a means of foreclosing on alternative realities—a way of defining the individual, delimiting the social, and managing the increasingly vexed and confusing relation between the two.[13]

Raw Material addresses a substantially different aspect of Victorian body politics, analyzing how the language of disease could frame the body not as the site of essential, inalienable human nature, but rather as a quantity of raw material, a malleable entity whose dumb bulk is inevitably molded—for better or for worse—in the very image of culture. Taking progressive disease as a kind of embodied allegory for social "progress," Victorian writers treated pathology as an absolutely material mode of fiction making, a system of signs that provided a means of anatomizing the problems and possibilities of industrial development. Symbolically disfiguring and transfiguring the body, the diseases I study here combined to develop something like a physiological relativism, a logic of embodiment whose understanding of human flesh as a dense, uncertain, deeply changeable material enabled it to rework the relationship between self and world. Pathology thus provided the basis for a kind of antiessentialist poetics, a means of imaginatively adapting to a culture wherein it was increasingly difficult to determine not only what it meant to be human, but also what it meant to be alive.

By looking at how Victorian signifying practices consistently make symptoms into signs, treating bodily process as the basis for narrative paradigms, this book aims to vex our present tendency to locate the material as a "real" outside of language. I take an intensely literary approach to nonliterary spaces (textual, visual, artifactual, corporeal), close reading their intersecting linguistic, anatomic, and imagistic patterns in order to illuminate how the unspeakable signs of disease—the ghastly ulcerations of cancer, the ghostly agonies of phantom limb pain—were pressed into the service of representation (phantom limbs took shape as somatic sensation fictions; cancerous breasts looked more like sewers than sexual organs). More specifically, I chart the mechanisms by which the diseased body's materiality—its pains, pus, sores, and even feces—was metaphorized at the same time that it remained irreducibly "real" (phantoms hurt; cancer kills). Concentrating on a series of moments when diseased and deformed flesh merges metaphorically with other things—when the exigencies of the material body are explained as problems of material culture—this book contends that nineteenth-century figurations of pathology constituted an elaborate meditation on the relationship between objects and persons: whether persons were objects; whether objects were subjects; and whether, and on what terms, there could be said to be any essential difference between the two.

In a world where things seemed to come alive, to have bodies and even minds of their own, and where bodies appeared to be increasingly stilted and mechanical, subordinated to the automotive requirements of machines, the problem of distinguishing between people and things was more than just an interesting philosophical question: it was a pressing and immediate concern. The first volume of Marx's *Capital* (1867) is perhaps the most famous articulation of how capitalism scrambles distinctions between bodies and objects by falsely animating things and fatally mechanizing workers.[14] However, Marx's account of material and mechanical threat must be seen as one of a series of competing narratives about materiality circulating during this time. The notion of bodies being overtaken or replaced by machines, for instance, was used toward a number of ideological ends. Industrial novels such as *Hard Times* (1854) and *Mary Barton* (1848) anticipate the trajectory of accounts like Marx's, arguing that because workers are irreducibly human they cannot survive a system that expects them to be machines—the "Hands" in Dickens's Coketown suffer precisely because they are not "only hands, or, like the lower creatures of the seashore, only hands and stomachs" (*Hard Times* 70). Other discourses, however, imagine mechanization as a means of securing an all-too-vulnerable humanity. As I go on to show in chapter 3, this is the operative fantasy of prosthesis, which imagines that the amputee's sense of himself as a whole man can be restored by merging his mangled limb with a machine.

As the example of prosthesis suggests, narratives that placed people and property in dynamic relation to one another, imagining that selves could intermingle with their stuff in mutually constitutive and enabling ways, were deeply compelling. To take just one example, Victorian writers developed an entire epistemology—even a psychology—of that quintessentially English artifact, the umbrella. The umbrella was seen to reflect, extend, and even complete its owner's personality: as an 1858 *Household Words* essay on "People's Umbrellas [as indices to character]" puts it, "This humble instrument is cherished as a street god—a companion—a something to hold silent communion with—an appendage which, like a dog or a walking-stick, is modified by the character of its owner, while it becomes, at the same time part of his system, exerting an influence over him equal to what it receives" (Hollingshead 496). This logic of material reciprocity, in which elemental and individual qualities cross over to create a perfect economy of character, appears over and over again in Victorian writing. Elsewhere in *Household Words*, Dickens describes his umbrella as a kind of phrenological prosthesis, a silken skull containing "all the best bumps in my head" ("Please to Leave Your Umbrella" 457), while "People's Umbrellas" depicts a nervous man's umbrella as an emotional wreck, an unstable structure with outbursts so powerful that it continually keels over and even occasionally wets itself. When propped up against the wall, "the ill-constructed nuisance opens with a burst and a splutter, falling helplessly in the little pool which it has deposited on the carpet" (Hollingshead 496). (There was help for such cases—a shop in Shoreditch advertised itself as an Umbrella Hospital, and, claiming to be able to do both physical and psychological repairs, charged sixpence for such minor services as "restoring a broken rib," "inserting a new spine," and supplying "new motive power," and one shilling for the more complex operations involved in "restoring a shattered constitution," "resuscitating the muscularia," "supplying a new head," and "supplying a new set of nerves" [Crawford 191].)[15] Taking on human features so completely that they seem to be, paradoxically, essential to their owners' sense of themselves as autonomous individuals, umbrellas embodied a fantasy of a world in which the massive proliferation of objects worked to solidify subjects, in which the least palpable qualities of being—taste, intelligence, frame of mind— could be materialized within the contours of things.

If personal property was seen as an extension of specific personalities, popular accounts of manufacture commonly attributed human qualities to raw materials. An 1850 *Household Words* essay entitled "A Paper-Mill" tells how rags are made into paper from the perspective of the materials—first rags, then pulp, and finally paper—themselves. Similarly, popular and technical accounts of vulcanization depict the refinement of india rubber as a civilizing process, a socialization of substance in which an exotic and unruly black mass is whitened, stabilized, and made into a range of socially useful products.[16] Together, these examples indicate the imaginative potential embedded within the epistemological and material confusions of machine culture, the sense that leveling constitutive distinctions between people and things enabled new models of identity and materiality to be conceptualized even as that leveling jeopardized distinctions among selves, their bodies, and the larger material world. This book situates pathology at the heart of this broad cultural dynamic. The physical alterations caused by disease made it possible to think more generally about the sheer malleability of human flesh—its capacity to be both displaced and replaced, violently destroyed and creatively remade by the newly industrial world. The body's capacity to be both melted down and molded in the image of the material environment in turn raised important questions about the essential nature of the modern Victorian self—about what it was, what it could be, and what it would have to become in order to survive the advent of technological modernity.

Raw Material is thus neither a history of Victorian medicine nor an analysis of the Condition of England; rather, it is an anatomy of a conjunction, a map of the metaphoric and material crossovers Victorians made between human bodies and industrial entities, between pathologies and emergent mass cultural processes. The stories I tell here about disease are consequently culled from, but not circumscribed by, narratives Victorians themselves framed—about disease, culture, bodies, things. Tracking metaphors, allusions, and images across a range of representational spaces, I break down boundaries between texts, disciplines, and genres in order to piece together strands of thinking that nowhere have a complete articulation, but which are present everywhere, albeit obliquely, in fragmentary, diffuse form. I have been principally concerned to see how, in the disparate spaces of medicine, literature, advertising, journalism, cartoons, photography—even body parts, gadgets, and dirt—certain clusters of images take shape, accumulating meaning as they recur across seemingly unrelated and disconnected texts, rather than through their orderly development within them. I have been concerned to uncover the stories the Victorians both were and were not telling, the meanings they were making in spite of themselves, the unwitting connections they were forging with overlapping metaphors, linguistic echoes, and conceptual metonymies. My goal has been to give shape to the accidental palimpsests of an inveterately verbal, and increasingly visual, culture; to assemble a particular series of hermeneutic loose ends into a coherent account of how an extraordinarily bizarre system of signification came into being. The logics I unravel here are interstitial ones, strange but consistent associations whose implications went largely unmarked by the culture that made them. Written in the margins of Victorian culture, this is ultimately a book about pattern; it is, in this respect, a study in the politics of adjacency, an attempt to assess the social significance of the Victorians' own substantial semiotic drift.

This wayward interpretive strategy yields new insights on both historical and methodological levels. On a historical level, it makes visible a correspondingly wayward picture of nineteenth-century identity formation. Much, if not all, of the work on Victorian selfhood concentrates on problems of subjectivity, equating the consolidation of bourgeois identity with the gradual emergence of the psychologically complex individual. Oddly enough, even explicitly materialist histories of the body such as Thomas Laqueur's *Making Sex* and Peter Stallybrass and Allon White's *Politics and Poetics of Transgression* end with Freud, as if to say that the natural conclusion to the madness of Victorian body politics is its sublation into hysterical speech. The goal of this project is to trace a strand of thinking that was separate from, and largely opposed to—if only by virtue of its sheer conceptual difference—master narratives of interiority. By looking at how Victorians used diseased bodies to think about beings as things (cities, sewers, novelties), *Raw Material* argues that pathology materialized a means of making and unmaking selves that neither presumed nor required a psychology. The stuff of a symbolic negotiation between competing ontologies of the physical, disease substantiated a series of allegories of objectification, varied accounts of material reduction, replacement, and reformation in which flesh is simultaneously broken down and built up into something else. The notion of disease as death by objectification (as in cholera and breast cancer)—or, conversely, the framing of disfigurement as a coming alive of the body as thing (as in prosthesis and the freak show)—encoded a problematic of material difference, a series of questions about how, and how much, the modern body "mattered." Those questions in turn constituted an elaborate meditation on the gendered, classed, and raced dimensions of the self in consumer society. The diseased body was symptomatic of the age: a focal point for both anxiety and exhilaration about the uncertain, shifting status of humanness in the age of capital, it imaged an emergent culture of surface, a world whose incipient modernity manifested itself not only in its penchant for making new identities, but also in its abiding fascination with watching itself make them.

These historical findings in turn provide the basis for a sustained investigation of the terms on which we currently write cultural history. In keeping with the book's effort to understand how it is that we come to read culture and write the past, each chapter takes on epistemological issues as well as historical ones, allowing primary material to generate methodological questions. Chapters 1 and 2 address problematic conceptual patterns in two prominent branches of contemporary cultural studies, showing the tendency for analogical thinking to overdetermine historical arguments in both postcolonial and feminist theory. Chapters 3 and 4, by contrast, work to historicize two of cultural studies' pet metaphors, showing how the "radical" theoretical gestures proposed by prosthesis and monstrosity are embedded in a distinctly conservative conceptual past. In each chapter, the nature of the evidence raises questions about how that evidence ought to be worked with. I address these questions along the way, integrating them into the analysis so as to reveal a series of connections between Victorian figurations of disease and contemporary critical paradigms. As such, the chapters talk to and through one another in necessarily contradictory ways: whereas the chapters on cholera and amputation are finally genealogies of contemporary theoretical concepts, the chapters on breast cancer and monstrosity call genealogical thinking into question by allowing epistemological similarities between Victorian models of culture and our own to demonstrate the practical impossibility of ever fully distinguishing between now and then. One of this volume's most pressing aims is thus to coax the "how" of its methods and the "what" of its materials into an ongoing dialogue. For it is only then that we may see how postcolonial theory's penchant for a language of contamination owes a conceptual debt to Victorian figurations of cholera as reverse colonization, or how nineteenth-century writing about breast cancer can actually provide a useful object lesson about the circulation of metaphor and synecdoche in cultural criticism. In so doing, *Raw Material* describes a past that grows more elusive the more it is written, and a present whose own investments in that past are as difficult as they are essential to grasp. As the title of the study indicates, *Raw Material* is finally about how knowledge is produced—not simply about how we shape the past into coherent stories, but about how the past has itself already shaped the terms on which we shape it.

Asiatic Cholera and the Raw Material of Race

This is the story of Asiatic cholera, as told by John A. Benson's 1893 treatise on the subject:

> Up from the dark Plutonian caverns of Erebus, up from the clouded Stygian valley, up from the depths of hell, in the early part of this century, arose the Goddess of Filth, and she wandered around over the face of the globe, seeking for a home to her liking. And coming to the delta of the Ganges, in this low, insalubrious and festering locality, where so many noxious and noisome diseases are generated, and where so many epidemics have arisen and so often swept over the earth with most fatal and desolating effects,—here she met, one dark and stifling night, with gaunt Despair. And surrounding her with his bony arms, Despair threw her on the foul, dark and slimy ground, and had his will of her. And when the day of her reckoning was reached, here in the neighborhood of Jessore—a town in the center of the delta—in agony and in shame and in desolation, Filth gave birth to the monstrosity yclept,—Asiatic cholera. And here she nurtured and fed him, here in this vast pest-house where every conceivable vegetable and animal substance is left upon the soil to rot in the heat and dews of a tropical climate,—here Filth fed her offspring from her own breasts, and as he grew and waxed strong, and his tusks and teeth

appeared so that he would chew and tear her dugs, she longed to wean him, and one day as he ferociously fastened himself upon her, she cast him away on the mud, and as his mouth was forcibly torn from the dug, some of her foul milk was scattered around, and falling into the water of the Ganges, as drops, was at once coagulated by the water, and became—the Spirilla Cholerae Asiaticae. (25)

In this epic invocation of the disease, Benson imagines the genesis of Asiatic cholera on the polluted banks of the Ganges as the result of a brutal environmental rape. The unwanted product of a hellish environment, the bastard child of "Filth" and "Despair," Asiatic cholera's is the case history of a criminal type. Describing an eerily Oedipal drama of epidemic, Benson envisions a psychology of infection in which the virulence of the disease results from being prematurely torn from the nurturing breast. Cholera, filled with anger at his mother, develops a kind of contagious character flaw, an unhealthy need to spread his devastation around. Born in 1817 in the Indian town of Jessore (about a hundred miles from Calcutta), cholera matured over the course of the 1820s into a marauder of "malignant character" (Jameson 167), an incompetent military commander whose circuitous route across Europe betrayed the backwardness of the world from which it came: "We never thought cholera would be so bad a general, with the example of Napoleon before his eyes, as to penetrate into the north of Europe, where, as we believed, like his great prototype, his force would be destroyed by frost and snow" ("The Contagious Character of Cholera" 123). Cruel and confused, a "monster" (Jameson 165) "truly of a protean nature" (Jameson 103), cholera's violence was all the more frightening for being totally unpredictable—"so diversified in its phases, so erratic in its general character, that it must be treated in its individuality" (Jameson 239), "choleraic perniciousness" was consistent only insofar as it habitually expressed itself in "deadly assaults" (Jameson 167) on the poor inhabitants of European cities.

Asiatic cholera took shape in the Victorian imagination as an Oriental raider, a barbaric force whose progress westward exposed the weak spots of an expanding industrial culture. According to the Canadian physician and health commissioner Robert Nelson, for example, Asiatic cholera is the most distinctive event of the nineteenth century:

The 19th century is remarkable for the great events that have taken place since its commencement, and a short time previously. In it the knowledge of steam, its powers, the means of controlling it, its uses as a substitute for bodily and manual labor, and its complete obedience to the hand of man, have been perfected.

Chemistry, already in its infancy, has become an exact science.

Electricity and magnetism have advanced from being mere toys to a grade of highest utility. Geology has disinterred the long buried almanac of the globe, brought clearly into light the reign of extinct creations, overwhelmed and hidden since millions of years have passed away. These are only a few of the remarkable occurrences; but the one which distinguishes this century more than all others of which history makes mention, in relation to man, is the stupendous plague called Cholera. Stupendous from its widespread malignancy over every continent; stupendous from the millions of victims it has swallowed; stupendous from the rapidity of its spread; stupendous from the few brief moments of life it allows to those it attacks: apparently capricious in its selections, it has desolated some places, spared others; terrified nations, arrested the march of armies, and baffled the efforts of man to arrest its empire. (13–14)

For Nelson, the most characteristic event of a century of progress is the emergence of an Oriental force capable of overthrowing the Western world; what symbolizes the industrial revolution more than any one technological event is the violent colonization of the West by an Eastern disease that is itself immune to the controlling powers of scientific modernity.[1] Imagining cholera as a kind of military invader, an infectious imperialist who not only destroyed lives but also dismantled the terms on which the West understood itself, Victorian physicians and social critics used the epidemic disease as a means of questioning how the West was securing its own global economic power.

Infecting all the filthiest spots of Europe and America, Asiatic cholera found a particularly hospitable home in the English slum, where it thrived amid the distinctive dirt of British streets. The great paradox of cholera was, indeed, its terrible power over the country that so thoroughly dominated its place of origin. An upstart Eastern infection that ought never to have come as far as it did, Asiatic cholera exposed the

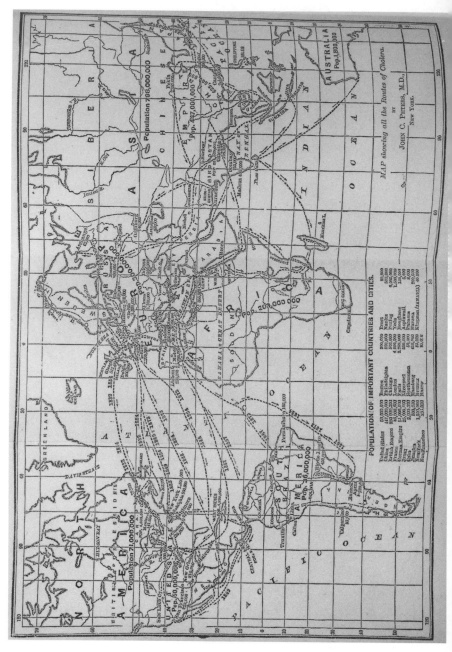

Fig. 1. The routes of cholera. From Edmund Charles Wendt, *Treatise on Asiatic Cholera* (1885). Courtesy of the College of Physicians, Philadelphia.

frailties of England's urban industrial structure, ravaging it on four separate occasions in as many decades. Cholera first showed itself on English shores in the shipping town of Sunderland in the fall of 1831, and over the next few months spread to Scotland, Manchester, the Midlands, and London. That outbreak killed around half of its victims, leaving 32,000 English subjects dead and thousands more devastated, destitute, and weak. Cholera struck again in 1848–49, killing 62,000; in 1853–54, killing 20,000; and again in 1866–67, killing 14,000 (Wohl 118).[2] Attacking the weak spots in the most powerful nation in the world with devastating accuracy and speed, cholera was seen as a sort of somatized social critique, a lethal disease whose pathological patterns provided a perfect map of the worst parts of England. Victorians developed an entire choleraic cartography, obsessively charting the course of the disease on global and local levels (figs. 1–3). A mystery to doctors and laymen alike, an exotic force that could neither be prevented nor cured and that killed with a speed and violence that was frightening to behold, it was a fitting figure for a culture that was ceasing to know itself, an inscrutable force from beyond that relentlessly exposed the underside of industrial development.

England's cholera years bracketed the period of deep uneasiness and ethical uncertainty that marked the early industrial decades of the Victorian period.[3] The years from 1831 to 1866 saw dramatic changes—the rise of the mass market and the beginning of the free trade era; the extension of the franchise to all propertied white men with the Reform Bill of 1832; the creation of a state-sponsored, punitive system of poor relief with the New Poor Law of 1834; the passage of a series of factory acts geared toward improving working conditions; and the birth of the public health movement (following the investigations of such men as James Phillips Kay, Edwin Chadwick, Thomas Southwood Smith, Neil Arnott, and William Farr, a centralized board of health was created in 1848). The population of cities tripled during the first half of the century, and modern transportation was born: tens of thousands of miles of railroad track were laid during the 1830s and 1840s, and in 1854 work on the London Underground began. Irish people immigrated to England, and English people emigrated to America by the thousands. A massive, politically aware urban underclass was formed; overseas markets were rapidly expanded; and after the Indian Mutiny of 1857, the

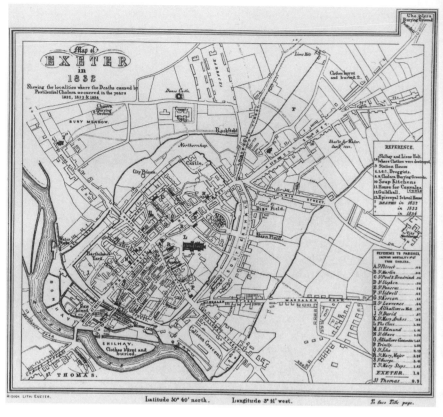

Fig. 2. Cholera map of Exeter in 1832. From Thomas Shapter, *The History of the Cholera in Exeter in 1832* (1849).

state assumed official control over India. Victorian writers capitalized on the historical convergence of economic growth and epidemic spread, using Asiatic cholera as a metonymy for the disruptive effects of social change. Over the course of the century, Asiatic cholera became a master trope for urban existence. Throughout Europe and North America, it was a figure for and function of the deep uncertainty of modern culture. Periodicals, newspapers, and broadsides pictured cholera everywhere: as a giant ravaging war-torn Europe, a vagabond walking the streets of revolutionary Paris, even as a half-rotten corpse en route to America. The popular press showed a screeching miasmatic cholera wafting through the air on waves of stench, and a magnified microbial cholera riding around on the backs of men, 125,000 times larger than life. A

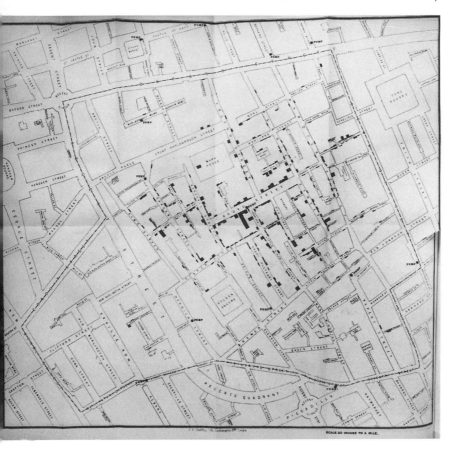

Fig. 3. Cases of cholera around the Broad Street pump during the 1854 epidemic in London. From John Snow, *On the Mode of Communication of Cholera* (1855). Courtesy of the College of Physicians, Philadelphia.

skeletal cholera pumped contaminated water for the poor, gave dinners for the damned, and even traveled to Spain, where it posed as a toreador taunting death itself.[4] Capable of assuming any form and dictating any number of meanings, cholera was a metaphor for it all, an absolutely embodied figure for the exigencies of existence in the age of capital. Linked in the popular imagination to such pervasive social problems as immigration, poverty, poor sanitation, and revolution, cholera was synonymous with the modern condition; it was everywhere and everything at once.

But for all its worldly ways, cholera reigned supreme in England. As

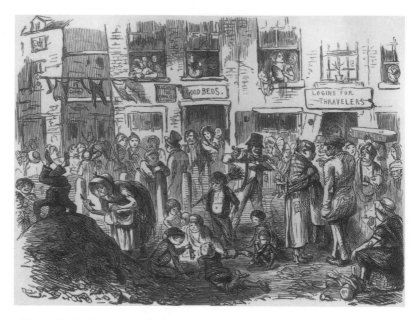

Fig. 4. Cholera's minions. From John Leech, "A Court for King Cholera," *Punch* (1852).

an 1852 *Punch* cartoon called "A Court for King Cholera" (fig. 4) indicates, cholera was the lord of English slums, and England was cholera's home away from home. From 1832 on, Asiatic cholera came to function as a kind of master referent in the Condition of England debate, a means of articulating concerns about the effect of the industrial revolution on the English self. Victorian writers continually coupled Asiatic cholera with the problems of urban culture in order to develop a thoroughgoing critique of the contemporary urban scene. Noting that cholera typically settled in slums—it was a disease "of a vagrant character" (quoted in Jameson 54) that had, "in his rambles," a "preference for mud and mire, and crowded houses, and low places" (Jameson 277)—nineteenth-century writers used the suggestive patterns of cholera's spread as the material of social critique, developing an entire narrative of corporeal conquest to signal the precariousness of national identity under capitalism. In the absence of satisfying scientific explanations for the spread of disease, British writers developed a poetics of contagion that juxtaposed invention and infection, progress and plague, industry and empire. In so doing, they combined anxieties about the condition of England into a socially resonant, powerfully evocative account of physical threat.

MAKING PLAGUE

In his influential *Treatise on Fever* (1830), the physician Thomas Southwood Smith develops a vocabulary of contagious manufacture to link the fetid, close conditions of English slums to the deadly atmosphere of Africa. Setting epidemic, exoticism, and industry in dynamic relation to one another, Smith figures infectious disease as a foreign commodity that is beginning to be duplicated successfully by domestic modes of production: "The room of a fever patient, in a small and heated appartment [*sic*] of London, with no perflation of fresh air, is perfectly analogous to a stagnant pool in Ethiopia, full of the bodies of dead locusts. The poison generated in both cases is the same; the difference is merely in the degree of its potency. Nature, with her burning sun, her stilled and pent-up wind, her stagnant and teeming marsh, manufactures plague on a large and fearful scale: poverty in her hut, covered with her rags, surrounded with her filth, striving with all her might, to keep out the pure air, and to increase the heat, imitates nature but too successfully; the process and the product are the same" (324). In English cities as in Ethiopian swamps, plague is made, or "manufactured," as a matter of course: "the process and product are the same." In Nature, however, the catalytic combination of hot sun and stagnant marsh enables disease to be mass-produced "on a large and fearful scale," while in London fever is as yet a relatively small cottage industry, the piecemeal production of cramped, airless rooms. Imagining the ubiquitous problem of "fever" as a distinctly exotic by-product of urban space, Smith positions the capacity to manufacture disease as a sign and a symptom of a particularly unfortunate industrial achievement: rather than importing plague, the English are making their own.[5]

   The notion that industrial England was manufacturing an environment uncannily akin to that of Smith's pathogenic African scene of "burning sun," "teeming marsh," and "stagnant pool" was a common one during the Victorian era. Exoticism provided a compelling metaphor for the effects of industrialism on the English environment, enabling commentators not only to emphasize how alien the urban landscape was, but also to align that apparent foreignness with filth and disease. According to an 1842 article in the *Quarterly Review*, for example, unsanitary conditions were effectively transforming parts of England into Africa, generating atmospheric poisons that in turn produced what appeared to be tropical disease: "It has been repeatedly observed that the family of a particular house has continued for years to be constantly afflicted with the very languor and fever described by every African traveler, which at last has been ascertained to have been caused by the introduction into the immediate neighbourhood of a couple of square feet of Sierra Leone, or, in plainer terms, by a grated untrapped gulley-drain, from which there has been constantly arising a putrid gas; and yet, instead of a few square feet, how many acres of Sierra Leone are, to our shame, existing at this moment in our metropolis in the shape of churchyards!" ("Report on the Sanitary Condition of the Labouring Classes" 422). By suggesting that urbanization produced living conditions that matched or even fell short of the "primitive" ones found abroad, comparisons such as this one worked to indicate that England, in consolidating its power as the strongest industrial nation in the world, was somehow ceasing to be English, that even as it was establishing imperial dominance over millions of exotic others, parts of it were becoming other to itself. Worried that the urban landscape was turning into "one of the strangest jumbles of artificial civilization and primeval barbarism which the world has ever beheld" (Kingsley, "The Water Supply of London" 124), social critics agreed that England was mass-producing a distinctly exotic squalor out of its own ill-disposed waste: as *Fraser's* put it in 1849, "The main difference is that *we make our own* swamps in England, and compensate for a hotter sun by fouler water, which water, let it not be forgotten, we drink" ("Cholera Gossip" 708; my emphasis).

From the moment of its arrival in England, Asiatic cholera was the primary figure in the Orientalist rhetoric of industrial filth. An Indian disease that flourished in English towns, Asiatic cholera materialized the figurative link that Smith and others made between exotic infection and urban conditions, providing palpable confirmation of the gross similarities between industrial and Oriental space. As *Fraser's* observed at the height of the 1849 outbreak, it was no mystery why cholera had sought out England a second time: "Let us not forget that the cholera of

1817, whatever may have been the history of its birth and parentage, had a swamp for its cradle, and poor Indian serfs, earning twopence half-penny a day, broiling under a vertical sun, and living, doubtless, as poor workmen live in more favoured lands, after a very miserable and squalid fashion, for its first victims. If we had conned this lesson well in 1832, we should not have had to record so many thousand deaths in 1849. We should have recognized in every part of England worse swamps than those of Bengal, and more likely victims than the Pariahs of Jessore" ("Cholera Gossip" 706). Thriving in the grubbiest courts and feeding on the plentiful bodies of the poor, Asiatic cholera became the focal point of a degenerative narrative of urban transformation, powerfully suggesting that in some respects England had become more Indian than India itself.[6] According to the *Westminster Review* in 1831, the English poor lived in worse conditions than Indians did: "In many respects no town which Cholera has yet visited, can furnish an easier conquest than our own metropolis. The hundreds of starving paupers who come to London for relief, and are compelled from want to herd together in much less cleanliness and comfort than the lowest orders of the native Indians, are ever predisposed to the invasion of such an epidemic" ("Spasmodic Cholera" 486).

As if to say that the poor were vulnerable to Asiatic cholera because they were Asiatic already, Victorian social criticism continually aligned the fact of infection with the fantasy of foreignness. If the poor were native pariahs, slathered in filth and aching with want, poor neighbor-hoods were themselves modernized Indias, the busy centers of a bar-baric manufacturing system. London in particular was likened to India time and time again—in an 1849 article on the sanitary conditions of Bermondsey, a particularly wretched London slum, Henry Mayhew calls the neighborhood of Jacob's Island the "very capital of cholera, the Jessore of London" (32). Other commentators located numerous Black Holes to rival Calcutta's notorious one.[7] The sanitary reformer Edwin Chadwick described the unventilated homes of the poor as urban ver-sions of the infamous Indian structure where 154 English prisoners suf-focated during a hellish night in 1756 (277); *Fraser's* wrote that the 1848 cholera outbreak at the boarding school at Tooting, where more than 200 of the 1,400 children died in the space of two weeks, was "unparal-leled since the days of the Black Hole at Calcutta" ("Cholera Gossip"

708); and in 1842 the *Quarterly Review* even compared the drawing rooms of wealthy houses to the stifling atmosphere of the Indian cell: during parties, the guests were "like those in the Black-hole at Calcutta, conglomerated together in a hermetically-sealed box full of vitiated air" ("Report on the Sanitary Conditions of the Labouring Classes" 419).[8] Breaking up London into a series of stagnant spaces where rich and poor alike smothered and gasped for air, Victorians relied on the legendary Indian hellhole as a point of sanitary reference, a means of forcefully demarcating one of the central paradoxes of "progress": that inhuman living conditions were the end result of "civilized" life. At once an Indian wasteland and an industrial center, England appeared to be mechanically reproducing the diseased environment of empire. As an Irish physician explained, "The fever nests have mysteriously and unaccountably become cholera nests. . . . The same raw materials have been used for the production of a totally new manufacture" (quoted in Longmate 168). The first truly new disease to reach the West since the sweating sickness of 1485,[9] Asiatic cholera was a thoroughly modern form of plague, the nation's newest, most feverish manufacture.

Statistically, Asiatic cholera was not the most lethal disease of the Victorian period. It killed far fewer people than endemic diseases such as fever, tuberculosis, measles, and influenza; indeed, in 1848 influenza killed fifty thousand people in London alone, more than five times the number that would die from cholera in that city the following year. Even so, cholera's social significance was tremendous; it killed with a violence that was shocking to behold, and no one knew what caused it or how it could be cured. But the disease itself was unmistakable: horribly dehydrated after purging massive amounts of "rice-water" diarrhea, its victims could be dead within a few hours and seldom lasted more than two or three days. So great was the impact of cholera on Victorian sensibilities that it inspired the first sociological investigations of slums and ultimately motivated a series of legislative and bureaucratic measures dedicated to sanitary reform; indeed, Asiatic cholera was in many ways directly responsible for the birth of the public health movement in Britain.[10] Lending substance to the Condition of England debate in a way endemic diseases never could, Asiatic cholera was *the* industrial epidemic, crowding other diseases out of the popular imagination almost as soon as it arrived. As early as 1832, the *Examiner* announced that cholera had moved in on fever's traditional turf: "Cholera takes up its abode in the haunts of fever; it has assumed the place of fever, because it has nearly banished it from the metropolis and has itself become the epidemic of the season" (quoted in Pelling 49). A "totally new manufacture," Asiatic cholera was the novel contagion of the nineteenth century, "the epidemic of the season," a side effect and a symbol of industrial culture, a brand-new disease that was all the rage. Condensing a range of anxieties about economic development into the symptomatology of cholera, Victorian writers combined epidemic and industry into a rhetoric of commodified contagion, a social fiction of spread in which pathology functioned as a metaphor for and commentary on the rise of commercial culture.

Thought by many to be transmitted by "infected goods" (Nelson 138), cholera was closely linked to material culture, associated with everything from mail (which could deliver "cholera dust"—deadly particles of dried-up diarrhea—to remote destinations) to musical instruments. One late-century medical treatise warned of the particular dangers of pianos, whose nooks, keys, pedals, and strings were impossible to disinfect thoroughly (Benson 215). More common, however, were concerns about the contagious powers of clothing, bedding, and food. Case reports tracking the transmission of disease via infected clothing and bedding abounded—cholera had been spread by the contents of a suitcase more than once ("after cholera matter has passed into the *dried* state, healthy men may carry it about in their baggage" [Peters 58]), and cases of washerwomen coming down with cholera after laundering the sheets and nightshirts of victims were commonplace. Additionally, doctors warned that certain foods rendered people especially vulnerable to invasion by disease—the "abuse of fruit," for instance, was thought to be a virtual invitation to infection ("Cholera Gossip" 703). Mayhew's street sellers felt the effects of such dietetic "choleraphobia," reporting that during the epidemic of 1849, the sale of potatoes, greens, fruit, and fish dropped off dramatically (*London Labour and the London Poor* 1:59).[11] Cholera was, of course, not the only source of infectious objects. England was rife with contagious commodities, and horror stories of how things could carry sickness from the hovels of the poor into the homes of the rich abounded. In an essay called "Cheap Clothes and Nasty," Charles Kingsley recounts a series of such cases in order to show

how all of society is damaged by the degraded conditions of the poor: "The Rev. D— finds himself suddenly unpresentable from a cutaneous disease, which it is not polite to mention on the south of Tweed, little dreaming that the shivering dirty being who made his coat had been sitting with his arms in the sleeves for warmth while he stitched at the tails. The charming Miss C— is swept off by typhus or scarlatina, and her parents talk about 'God's heavy judgment and visitation'—had they tracked the girl's new riding-habit back to the stifling, undrained hovel, where it served as a blanket to the fever-stricken slopworker, they would have seen *why* God had visited them" (98).[12] Cholera occupied a special place in this broad social uneasiness about the potential of goods to link different types of people through shared infection, dramatizing a material connection not only between hardship and luxury (the problem with contagious pianos, for example, was that they brought cholera out of the rookeries and into the drawing room), but also narrowing the gulf between East and West.

Popularly understood as an "imported infection" (Creighton, *History* 2:819), Asiatic cholera took shape as an inherently exotic commodity, an object that, for all its contact with English things, was always already infected by the East.[13] Like the foreign products that flooded English markets during the nineteenth century, cholera was a strange and unfamiliar thing fresh from the Orient. Writers capitalized on this overlap between economic trends and patterns of epidemic spread, treating Asiatic cholera as both a symptom and a side effect of England's increasing interest in the raw materials and manufactures of empire.[14] The patterns of cholera's spread absolutely paralleled those of importation. One treatise noted that it "follows the lines of human traffic, progressing along the world's most frequented highways, with a rate of speed that is in direct ratio with that afforded by the means of human intercommunication" (Benson 78). Another noted that, like a shipment of goods, cholera's rates of travel over land and sea were carefully logged: "When it reached Europe in 1830, it traveled from eighty to one hundred miles a week, and crossed the Atlantic, in old-fashioned sailing-vessels, at a speed of three or four hundred miles in seven days" (Peters 30). So firmly was cholera linked to trade that even the language used to describe its actions in the body contained references to it. One medical treatise explained the fragility of the cholera bacillus, which could not thrive in an environment populated by other microorganisms, as a form of economic instability: Asiatic cholera was "a 'protective tariff' bacillus" that could "not compete with foreign labor" (Benson 63). Packed up in boxes and wrapped in cloth, following the major trade routes across Europe to England with unprecedented speed, cholera was a thoroughly modern plague, a scourge whose spread was modulated by the demands of an emergent mass market for the spices and silks of the East.[15] Taking up residence in the neighborhoods of the poor just as more benign imports began to make their way into the parlors of the middle class, cholera was the poor man's novelty, the piece of the East that every Englishman, however humble, could acquire.

Cholera not only charted the course of a growing global economy, it also incorporated the queasiness of cultural shift in its very symptoms. The initial stages of infection, for instance, were described as the onset of a distinctly modern malaise. According to a pamphlet issued by a regional board of health in 1831, the first phase of cholera was a whirlwind experience, a rapid-fire succession of intensely unfamiliar feelings: "If the attack occurs in the day, the patient sits down affrighted at his own situation; or if in bed awakes and lies for a moment astonished at the novelty of his feelings; there is a new influence that appears to pervade the whole of his body" (quoted in McLaughlin 140). Expressing itself as a series of "novel feelings" and "new influences," cholera was typical of a century that prided itself on its seemingly infinite capacity to generate novelty. As an 1863 advertising manual noted, newness was the defining feature of modern life: "there is nothing under the sun now that is *not* new. Novelty is the order of the day" (W. Smith 7). Fast paced and violent, packing a world of feeling into its symptoms, Asiatic cholera was a kind of autonomic adventure. Like the disorienting plenty of the department store, the nerve-wracking effects of sensation fiction, or the giddy speed of the railroad, cholera caused a sensational vertigo that reproduced in concentrated form the frenetic feel of modernity.

Victorians kept up a running commentary on the special stress of modern life. Neurosis, neurasthenia, depression, and fatigue were all diagnoses that indicated the "human motor's" inability to cope with the pace and pressure of modern existence.[16] Everyone suffered at times from stretched, frayed, or shattered nerves, telling signs of overextended lives. And the sense of having worn inner workings led people to complain of being "spent," "drained," and otherwise reduced by daily experience. Charles Dickens, for example, was fatigued into total confusion by the Great Exhibition of 1851: "I find I am 'used up' by the Exhibition. I don't say there is nothing in it: there's too much. I have only been twice, so many things bewilder one. I have a natural horror of sights, and the fusion of so many sights in one, has not decreased it" (quoted in Gibbs-Smith 26). The onset of cholera mimicked the uneasiness of such sensory overload. Overwhelmed by the sheer volume of novel sensations—the "fluttering in the pit of the stomach," the "sense of weight or constriction round the waist," the "prickly sensation in the arms and legs, extending sometimes to the fingers and toes," the "copious clammy moisture" of hands and feet, the "suppressed and slow" pulse, and the "pain in the forehead"—the cholera victim suffered something like the characteristic collapse of consumer culture, the extravagant exhaustion of redundant experience (quoted in McLaughlin 140–41). Bewildered and depleted—indeed, completely dehydrated—by the extremity of the experience, by the "fusion" of so many sensations in one, victims could neither assimilate nor fathom the danger those symptoms represented.[17] Putting the body through more than the mind could take in (one of the horrors of cholera was that victims remained fully alert as they rapidly wasted away), cholera condensed the confusions of mass culture into a current of change in which unsuspecting victims could be carried away almost before they knew they were going to be ill. Asiatic cholera was a physiological too-muchness that literally stopped people in their tracks (it was not uncommon for victims to be struck down in the streets). Marked at first "only by a sudden uneasiness" (Tardieu 7), cholera internalized in devastating fashion the nervous dis-ease of modernity itself.[18]

The broad similarity between the novelty of cholera and the nausea of commodity culture is typical of writing about the disease, which routinely compressed the diffuse impressions of modern life into cholera's distinctive series of symptoms. At its height as a social threat when the Great Exhibition of 1851 ushered in the era of high capitalism, cholera coincided with the rise of consumer culture, and as such it became the means of expressing deeply felt anxieties about social change.[19] Im-

ported from India and manufactured at home, Asiatic cholera captured
the rhythms of a rapidly altering culture, compressing the changed,
changing character of contemporary existence into a violent trajectory
of illness. If the first phases of cholera replicated the sickening delir-
ium of urban experience, the later stages of the disease incorporated a
series of nightmarish tableaux of industrial life. Asiatic cholera was a
corporeal form of culture shock, a paranoid physiology whose characteristic diarrhea flowed into widespread fears of personal dissolution,
and whose final phase of dehydrated collapse fostered fantastic sce-
narios of a regressive reduction of the self to so much raw material.

WASTING AWAY

Much Victorian writing about the effects of industrialism on the national health figures Asiatic cholera as a crucial vector, an infectious
index of the well-being of English society.[20] Sir John Simon's 1854
report on the nature of "cholera poison" makes the barometric function
of Asiatic cholera abundantly clear, arguing that the disease is less a malignant force in itself than a measure of the malignancy of urban space:

> That which seems to have come to us from the East is not itself a
> poison, so much as it is a test and touchstone of poison. Whatever in
> its nature it may be, this at least, we know of its operation. Past
> millions of scattered population it moves innocuous; through the
> unpolluted atmosphere of cleanly districts it migrates silently with-
> out a blow,—that which it can kindle into poison lies not there. To
> the foul damp breath of low-lying cities it comes like a spark to
> powder. Here is contained that which it can swiftly make destruc-
> tive,—soaked into soil, stagnant in water, grimming the pavement,
> tainting the air,—the slow rottenness of unremoved excrement, to
> which the first contact of this foreign ferment brings the occasion of
> changing into new and more deadly combinations. (Quoted in "Mr.
> Simon's Report," *Littell's Living Age* 428)[21]

For Simon, as for many others, patterns of choleraic contagion encoded
a kind of sickening social commentary, exposing the deadly nature of
city life by "kindling" the "poisons" that were lying latent in the filthy
corners and fetid air of the great towns. Positing an excremental affinity

between East and West, writers like Simon saw cholera as a catalyst for the inherent pathology of metropolitan culture—as Simon explains in his report, the incidence of cholera "mainly varies with the degree in which a dense population lives in the atmosphere of its own excrement" (quoted in Newton v). Binding East and West together in a common problematic of filth, excrement made palpable the view that England was deteriorating into a distinctly Oriental compost of human waste.

India was itself famous for its magnificent filth, especially for its peculiar and unhealthy tolerance of human and animal waste. According to one medical treatise, Indians display the "utmost recklessness as to the disposal of all descriptions of offal, and more particularly of the dejections from the human intestine. . . . [T]he filth of the native villages requires to be seen to be believed in; and the streets of all the cities are narrow, dirty, and ill-paved" (Peters 11). Another observes that "the people are naturally devoid of habits of cleanliness, and almost of decency; if allowed, they will not only resort to the public thoroughfares for the purposes of nature, but will construct cloacae under the rooms in which they lie, cook, and sleep" (quoted in Peters 11). The notorious dirt of India became a point of sanitary reference for social critics, who worried openly about the fact that England was itself awash in waste. An 1850 article in the *Quarterly Review* gives voice to this excremental anxiety, observing that "it is, indeed, curious to note the hidden relations between private and public cleanliness; relations, not merely connecting the defecation of our own dwellings with that of London at large; but even making our personal ablutions, and the general scavenging of the town, part and parcel of the same operation" ("Sanitary Consolidation" 482). Expressing its belief in a fecal contamination of city space, the essay charts the movement of this contamination, tracking its progress from the bowels to the sewers through the streets, watching as it dries and swirls through the atmosphere and finally spirals into the lungs, back to the bodies whence it came. Countless essays and reports on sanitary conditions combine to tell a singular story of cultural contamination, a rank tale of how millions of closely packed urban bowels were producing a huge fecal backlog, a defecatory excess in which the uncollected and ill-disposed waste of cities clogged drains, sat in sewers, piled up in privies, soaked through walls, saturated the water supply, paved the streets, and even lined the lungs. When droppings on the street dry up, they form dark, rank "dust-clouds" that "are deposited on our clothes and furniture; on our skins, our lips, and on the air-tubes of our lungs. . . . [T]here is not at this moment a man in London, however scrupulously cleanly, nor a woman, however sensitively delicate, whose skin, and clothes, and nostrils, are not *of necessity* more or less loaded with a compound of powdered granite, soot, and a still more nauseous substance" ("Sanitary Consolidation" 482–83). In the excremental imagination of Victorian culture, this "nauseous substance" binds private and public space as the municipal inability to cope with the voluminous movements of its population creates an entire fecal topography.

In his *Sanitary Ramblings,* the urban explorer Hector Gavin maps a festering geography of city streets, describing the accumulated dirt of Bethnal Green as substantial geological formations. On Digby St. Globe Road, for instance, "a person named Baker, lately dead, here formed a receptacle for every kind of manure. The premises have a frontage of 450 feet, and are about 140 feet in depth. With the exception of a small space in front, and on either side, the whole of the area is filled with every variety of manure in every stage of offensive and disgusting decomposition; the manure is piled up to a considerable height, and is left to dry in the sun; but, besides this table mountain of manure, extensive and deep lakes of putrefying *night soil* are dammed up with the more solid dung, and refuse, forming together, mountain and lake, a scene of the most disgusting character" (9). Pleasant Place offers by contrast a more aquatic prospect, "nothing more or less than an elongated lake or canal; only, in place of water, we have a black, slimy, muddy compost of clay and putrescent animal and vegetable remains" (11); while Hague Street is a kind of urban bottom: "There is a large and deep hollow, in the shape of an irregular triangle, with the sides measuring respectively about 130, 130, and 100 feet. In wet weather this is a sort of pond; into it are thrown at all times the contents of the fish-baskets, the heads and intestines of fish, and every kind of animal and vegetable refuse" (23). For Gavin, "night soil" and "more solid dung" form the topsoil of a sublime wasteland, building up into an overwhelmingly fetid landscape of mountainous manure, streaming sewage, and even offal ponds stocked with the discarded remains of dead fish.

Choleraic diarrhea was the master referent for these figurations. The primary signifier in the social semiology of excrement, it utterly liquidated the already muddy boundary between corporeal and civic space. In the minds of physicians and social commentators alike, the choleraic body and the city were coextensive, systems of ducts and drains that were run together by the turbid diarrhea of the cholera victim himself. Shooting out gallons of fluid that, like the London water supply, was clouded with foreign matter, the choleraic body in turn became a signifier for faulty sewerage, a network of pipes and pumps whose "fixtures [are] tarnished, cracked, and broken," allowing "unwonted products [to] accumulate" and "break[ing] up the works that are proper and necessary to be done" (Jameson 30). "Shut[ting] up normal outlets, and mak[ing] sluices of those that should be shut" (Jameson 277–78), cholera stopped up veins (tacky, dried-up blood could not flow), opened unsightly drains (oozing from the pores was a characteristic sign of collapse), and turned mouth and anus into a veritable waterworks: "The patient has from fifteen to twenty dejections, or even more, in the twenty-four hours. They escape in some fatal cases by an involuntary and almost continuous jet" (Tardieu 11–12). Pouring forth in "jets or spirts [*sic*]" (Tardieu 13), choleraic evacuations flowed better than the public pumps, whose feculent trickle was available only irregularly, at certain times of the day, on certain days of the week—"the bowels are emptied by a gush, with a squashing sound into the vessel, as water from a pump" ("M. Culloch and MacLaren on Cholera" 24). Cholera flushed one victim so thoroughly that his rectum "gurgled" as the last drops of fluid dribbled away (Tardieu 12). Not all bowels were so thorough, however. On postmortem, some resembled a sickish sink, a reservoir for what looked like domestic slops—"a liquid of the color of coffee to which milk has been added" (Jackson 10); "white ropy fluid, semi-transparent, resembling the white of eggs" (Jackson 31); "small masses like broken boiled rice" (Jackson 35); "livid red turbid liquid" like "the lees of wine" (Jackson 35); "a solid form . . . resembling exactly, both in color and consistence, boiled and chopped spinage [*sic*]" (Jackson 50); "coffee grounds" (Jameson 96); and even apple jelly: one colon was spread with "a thick yellowish grey mucus, like a 'marmelade de pommes'" (Jackson 72). Other bodies contained more pedestrian forms of sludge: bladders "full of muddy urine" (Jameson 47), and intestines corroded with everything from grit ("a watery mixture of dark brick-dust" [Jackson 50]) to slime ("numerous brownish flakes, resembling moss under water" [Jackson 21]) to nonspecific grime ("dirty, blackish fluid, resembling the scrapings of the gutter" [Jameson 178]). Full of the dust and droplets of London life, the muck of kitchens and the mire of streets, cholera corpses incorporated on a bodily level the sanitary emergency of the modern city. As the physician William Budd explained, the sewer is "a direct continuation of the diseased intestine" (quoted in Bynum 81).

Cholera thus became the operative term in an entire metaphorics of bodily contamination, a figure for the fluidity of boundaries in metropolitan space. If the choleraic body was an unsanitary city, the unsanitary city was dying of cholera. Poorly kept city pipes could even suffer a fate similar to that of the cholera victim: "House-drains [could] get choked with a pitchy coagulum—like the stagnant blood in a cholera-patient's veins" ("Sanitary Consolidation" 472). And just as choleraic diarrhea resembled city water, city water was full of pathogenic waste. London water was notoriously impure, a turbid swill that frequently tasted "as if putrefied . . . often contain[ed] worms an inch long," and was, according to many, "only fit to rinse a pail or cleanse the privy" (quoted in Kingsley, "The Water Supply of London" 121–122). Full of mosses and microscopic life, vegetable matter and fleshy bits (eels, living and dead, sometimes issued from taps, as did shrimps), the water supply was essentially a diluted form of sewage, an unfiltered solution that fed you, among other things, your own fecal remains. On drinking, "you are literally filled with the fruit of your own devices, with rats and mice and such small deer, paramecia, and entomostraceae, and kicking things with horrid names, which you see in microscopes at the Polytechnic, and rush home and call for brandy—without the water—with stone, and gravil [sic], and dyspepsia, and fragments of your own muscular tissue tinged with your own bile" (Kingsley, "The Water Supply of London" 229). Debates about water purification consequently centered not on whether the water was full of human waste—that was unanimously conceded—but on whether such water was safe to drink. As one particularly rabid critic of the Thames water wrote, "A slender portion of common sense . . . authorizes me to affirm, that a stream which receives daily the evacuations of a million human beings, of many thousand animals, with all the filth and refuse of various offensive manufactories . . . cannot require to be analyzed, except by a lunatic, to determine whether it ought to be pumped up as a beverage for the inhabitants of the Metropolis of the British empire" (quoted in Hamlin 89).[22] During epidemics, the city pipes ebbed and flowed with an especially deadly decoction: brimming with the evacuations of thousands of cholera victims, the water was, to say the least, unsafe to drink.[23]

Filtering through choleraic diarrhea diffuse concerns about the unhealthy publicity of urban bodily functions, Victorians used the symptomatology of epidemic disease to express their gut reactions to the dissolutions of modern life. A novel experience that essentially turned people inside out, Asiatic cholera was a graphic model of personal disintegration, living proof of the violence and speed with which the self could be overwhelmed and washed away by the current of change. In *The Condition of the Working Class of England* (1945), Engels argues that towns break up individuals by crushing their bodies together: the "colossal centralization" of cities, their "heaping together of two and a half millions of human beings at one point," ends in the "dissolution of mankind into monads"; the more people are crowded "ever closer and closer together," the more they become divided, cut off from each other and separated even from themselves. Imagining England as a busy urban jumble, "masses of buildings" and "human turmoil" all rolled into one, Engels depicts the problem of identity in urban space as one of self-possession: the barest glimpse of London's shores is "so vast, so impressive, that a man cannot collect himself, but is lost in the marvel of England's greatness before he sets foot upon English soil" (36–37). Similarly, Victorian novels are full of images of human obliteration, lost souls and pressurized selves who have been variously crushed and cracked open: in *Oliver Twist* (1837), Bill Sikes beats the prostitute Nancy to a pulp; in *Dombey and Son* (1844–46), Mr. Carker is smashed by a train and smeared along the tracks; in *Bleak House* (1853), Krook spontaneously combusts; and in *Our Mutual Friend* (1864–65), Bradley Headstone's head splits off from his body and floats through the city streets on its own. Like Engels's shattered citizen or the pulverized, mutilated, and exploded characters that populate Dickens's fiction, Asiatic cholera encapsulated a violent fantasy of physical annihilation, a sordid somatic vision of a self that had been spread too thin.

MAKING BLACK

When twelve-year-old Isabella Hazard was seized with violent diarrhea and searing muscle cramps during the early morning hours of October 17, 1831, her mother expressed a concern for what these symptoms were doing to her daughter's coloring. "What makes the child so black?" she asked the doctor as her daughter died, shrunken, shriveled, and dark. Isabella Hazard's doctor did not know what "made" his patient "so black," but after William Sproat, a sixty-year-old keelman, died with similar symptoms two days later, the medical community of Sunderland declared the reason: Asiatic cholera had reached England from the East. Blackening was a characteristic side effect of Asiatic cholera, which left even the wizened bodies of survivors a mottled surface of dry, dark skin: "The skin assumes a blue or blackish hue, which is almost general; the nails become livid and almost black, the fingers wrinkled, and the genital organs retracted. The volume of the body diminishes rapidly and perceptibly" (Tardieu 8).[24] Blackened and reduced, their cramped limbs twisted into rigid postures, victims of Asiatic cholera gave the appearance of having undergone a sort of pathological regression, a morbid devolution into monstrous shadows of their former selves. Depicting Asiatic cholera as a kind of biological warfare, medical and popular accounts of infection emphasized the transformative violence of the disease with a metaphorics of miscegenation, a penetrative model of pathology that saw victims as infected with blackness itself. Epidemic disease was imagined as a military conquest. The "invasion of the patient" (Nelson 80) was typically "viewed as a sort of warfare" (Jameson 136); "armed with 'fire and sword,' and arrows to pierce, poison to sicken, screws to twist the nerves, massy weights to crush the muscles" (Jameson 277), cholera pillaged the victim's body, and it also raped: "the first step in the disease is an orgasm" of the alimentary canal (Peters 84); the subsequent evacuations gave off "an insipid spermatic odour" as they drained away (Tardieu 8). Settling in "colonies" in the intestines, the "culture" of cholera took shape as a kind of contagious colonization, an exotic infection that spread savagery itself (Benson 52). The dusky corpses of cholera victims were even discussed in explicitly ethnological terms. Like the Negro, whose veins were popularly supposed to contain "black blood" (Lynn 587),[25] the veins and vital organs of the cholera victim were "engorged with black blood" (Coventry 70): livers in particular were seen at postmortem to be full of "much clammy, black blood" (Jameson 41), while the brain itself was typically "stuffed with black thick blood" (Jameson 62). As a consequence, the cholera victim was as darkly exotic as the African himself: "Look at the skin, and you might almost imagine you have an Ethiopian" (Jameson 282). And like the Ethiopian, popularly imagined to be a type of ape, the cholera victim bore a striking similarity to simian forms: he resembled a "monkey rather than a man" (quoted in Longmate 18).[26]

An epidemic disease that could "make" thousands of white working-class bodies "black," cholera lent itself to the development of a materially embodied fiction of collective vulnerability, a physiological fable in which squalid urban living enables the poor to be infected with a deadly dose of darkness. Striking the working-class populations of towns almost exclusively, and making them over in the image of the exotic Other, Asiatic cholera suggested a series of affinities between poverty and primitivism, a cultural likeness between urban and exotic space that expressed itself through a symptomatics of racial regression. As such, the discourse of Asiatic cholera worked to question the healthiness of England's massive economic growth. As if to say that cholera could generate a sort of pathological speciation, Victorian writing about the disease treated it as a form of manufacture, a morbid mode of production in which race itself was made.[27]

Cholera was, in this respect, part of a larger trend in Victorian social criticism, which routinely linked primitivism and production into a singular problematic of urban degeneration. The idea that the working class amounted to a world apart from England was developed by writers of various political leanings, who tended almost uniformly to depict workers as belonging to an alien culture, or even another race. Poverty was seen as a degenerative force that resulted in a distinctly urban form of bestiality, a brutish insensibility to filth, stench, cold, and want that was uniquely fitted to survival in the slum. As the *Edinburgh Review* explained it, "the neglected refuse of civilisation has the faculty of nourishing social savages among mankind, just as it provides the favourite haunts of the vermin which frequent sewers and dung heaps" ("Sanitary Reform" 216); "families have been found, even in London, huddling together like animals, the very instincts of humanity obliterated, and, like the brutes, relieving every want, and gratifying every passion in the full view of the community" ("Supply of Water to the Metropolis" 387). Coupling economic privation and ethnic alteration, such accounts figure the effects of poverty on slum dwellers as a form of social speciation by describing paupers as primitive types—a "race of pygmies" (Engels 168), "social savages," or, in the case of the Irish, "white chimpanzees" (Kingsley, *Letters* 107).[28]

Taking shape as an elemental form of racial transformation, cholera lent scientific substance to the widely voiced fear that industrial capitalism was mass-producing a separate world, that it was making a race of savages out of the raw material of the English working class. Indeed, mid-Victorian theories of the chemistry of race had much in common with the physiology of cholera. According to an 1857 article in *Household Words* entitled "Why Is the Negro Black?" black skin results from a failure of the liver to cleanse the body of excess haematin, the iron-based molecule responsible for the peculiarly metallic smell and taste of blood: "A hot climate disturbs the normal action of the blood; also of the liver. The imperfect oxygen accompanying great heat not only adds to the darkness of the arterial blood, but also, by the want of energetic respiration which it involves, tends to the over fatness and torpidity of the liver. By this inaction of the great cleansing agent, the haematin of the blood-cells accumulates in the system; and, wandering restlessly about, having no place to go to, and no business there at all, it gradually takes refuge and makes its settlement in the lower and spherical cells of the cuticle: which it thus bronzes, from orange-tawny down to negro black, according to the heat of the climate, the consequent inactivity of the liver, and the amount of haematin left as refuse in the system" (Lynn 587–88). Imagining dark skin as a kind of industrial accident—the result of a breakdown of "one of the most important wheels in our internal machinery" (587)—the author develops an entire metallurgy of race, a theory of color that explains blackness as a form of biological bronzing and extends its claims even to northern native populations, whose "copper-coloured skin" speaks to a similar process of somatic smelting: "Cold checks the action of the liver equally with heat; and the shivering Esquimaux owes, to his wretched fare and sluggish circulation, his social misery and natural desolateness, the excess of haematin which dyes his skin" (588). Materialist theories of racial differentiation figure blackness as a sort of industrial disease, the flawed product of the body's inability to process its own raw materials, and as such they explain the racial connotations of cholera. After all, the darkness of the cholera body is due to a buildup of iron: blood that has been drained of its fluid contents is thick and dark, composed almost entirely of hematin. The physiology of cholera thus embodies a mineralized model of racial production, darkening the body by bronzing it—"the dark color of the blood produces a blue or bronzed hue of those parts in which the thinness of the skin permits its color to be seen" (Peters 80)—or by converting it to lead: the skin often has a "leaden hue" (Coventry 63; Nelson 109).[29]

Such crossovers between industrial process and racial production were the stuff of popular motif as well as scientific inquiry. In Dickens's *Dombey and Son* (1844–46), for example, the lovesick Mr. Toots imagines not only that race could be manufactured, but that doing so would mechanically reconfigure race relations as romance: overcome by a desire to serve the woman he loves, he dreams of being "dyed black, and made Miss Dombey's slave" (632). Wilkie Collins's 1872 novel *Poor Miss Finch* puts still another spin on the subject, depicting the side effects of silver nitrate, a specific for epilepsy, in terms of racial conversion: when used to prevent seizures, silver nitrate leaves the skin a "devilish . . . coloring of livid blackish-blue" (167).[30] Where Victorian fiction linked race and raw material through such widely varied rubrics as love and medicine, Victorian social criticism developed an entire semiology of industrial dirt, a grimy model of racial production that makes the grubby deposits of industrial filth into the essential stuff of race. According to Henry Mayhew, prolonged contact with filth could effect a sort of racial transformation—dirt debases and dehumanizes, altering body chemistry along Asiatic lines. In a letter to the *Morning Chronicle* in September 1849, Mayhew describes his visit to the cholera districts of Bermondsey in terms of an Oriental geography of disease. Noting that "London would almost admit of being mapped out pathologically, and divided into its morbid districts and deadly cantons," he concentrates his attention on "the ward of cholera," where 6,500 of the 12,800 deaths from cholera over the past three months had occurred. At the heart of the cholera ward is Jacob's Island, the "very capital of cholera, the

Jessore of London"; "bounded on the north and east by filth and fever, and on the south and west by want, squalor, rags and pestilence," Jacob's Island epitomizes Mayhew's image of an English India, or an Indian England, an environment whose filth causes an exotic change in the inhabitants' complexions. Boasting an open sewer full of "green rotting weed" and the "swollen carcasses of dead animals, almost bursting with putrefaction," piles of rotting refuse, and "open doorless privies that hang over the water" leaving "dark streaks of filth down the walls where the drains from each house discharge themselves into the water," Jacob's Island is producing a sickly strain of people: "The inhabitants themselves show in their faces the poisonous influence of the mephitic air they breathe." Some are made pale by the ill effects of the atmosphere—"their skins are white, like parchment, telling of the impaired digestion, the languid circulation, and the coldness of the skin peculiar to persons suffering from chronic poisoning"—while others develop a hectic flush and glassy eyes, "showing the wasting fever and general decline of the bodily functions." Still others display a "brown, earthlike complexion," the appropriately exotic result of the Eastern atmosphere in which they live: their "sunk eyes, with the dark areolae round them, tell you that the sulphuretted hydrogen of the atmosphere in which they live has been absorbed into the blood" (31–34). Knee-deep in excrement ("the privies were full to the seat" [36]) and forced to drink the very water they defecate into (one little girl "dangled her tin cup as gently as possible into the stream [while] a bucket of night-soil was poured down from the next gallery" [37]), the poor of Bermondsey are declining into a dark-skinned people, dirty and diseased.

In Mayhew's account, the foul emanations of the atmosphere poison the blood and darken the skin; in other accounts, dirt itself doubles as the raw material of race. This kind of metonymic metamorphosis, in which dirty surfaces alter bodily substance, is most dramatic in the case of people whose work brings them into close contact with black material. Chimney sweeps, for example, seem to become increasingly simian in aspect as their skin is stained by soot. In Charles Kingsley's *Water Babies* (1863), dirt is linked to devolution as soot savages the sweep, making the "little, black, ragged figure" into "a small black gorilla" (25), "a jolly little black ape instead of a boy, with four hands instead of two" (36). Likewise, Charles Lamb's rhapsodic 1823 account of the darkling

aspect of young sweeps sees the sign of professional experience—dirt—
through the lens of racial transformation. As if degrees of difference
could be reckoned in superficial smudges, Lamb imagines the layers of
soot on a young sweep's face to be a record of his constitutional conversion from white boy to black: "I like to meet a sweep—understand me,
not a grown sweeper—old chimney-sweepers are by no means attractive—but one of those tender novices blooming through their first
nigritude, the maternal washings not quite effaced from the cheek"
(quoted in Mayhew, *London Labour and the London Poor* 2:366). Taking
the partial blackening of the young sweep's skin as an exotic mark of
professional nubility, Lamb reads the first cheeky flush of "nigritude" as
the sign of his laborious coming of age.

As if to say that black raw materials could make workers black, social
critics developed a Lamarckian conception of racial manufacture, a
substantive model of speciation in which the worker's dirty body is
transformed into so much "savage" material. Lamb saw sweeps as both
spots of soot—"dim specks," "poor blots"—and indigenous tribesmen—
"young Africans of our own growth"; combining the characteristics of
the noble savage with the less distinguished, indeed indistinct, properties of English waste, they are "innocent blacknesses," childlike bodies
of black stuff (quoted in Mayhew, *London Labour* 2:366). Similarly, the
home of one of Mayhew's grubbier sweeps was so sooty that its contents
had blurred into a series of strangely animalistic inkblots—"every person and every thing which met the eye, even to the caps and gowns of
the women, seemed as if they had just been steeped in Indian ink . . .
[one] savage was intoxicated, for his red eyes flashed through his sooty
mask" (2:368). Disease only accelerated this process of material devolution. One ailing mining family was melded into a sticky black lump:
"When the small-pox was prevalent in this district, I attended a man,
woman, and five children, all lying ill with the confluent species of that
disorder, in one bed-room, and having only two beds amongst them.
The walls of the cottage were black, the sheets were black, and the
patients themselves were blacker still; two of the children were absolutely sticking together" (quoted in Chadwick 316). Taking on the characteristics of race and raw material at the same time, the dirty bodies
of the poor acquired in this discourse a distinctly industrial ethnicity,
a prefabricated primitivism in which men and women were stamped

out in a machine-made image of blackness. (Some were even stamped out in the image of black machines. Mayhew describes a sweep who blended into the blackness of his mechanical sweeper: the "matted hair" of the "savage" sweep "looked as if it had never known a comb, [and] stood out from his head like the whalebone ribs of his own machine" [2:368]).[31] Imagining a world where race reveals itself in the blots, lumps, spots, and stains of working-class culture, Victorians pictured a humanity profoundly destabilized by dirt. Savagery, it seems, could be produced from the smudges of stuff, and race itself could rub off—or on.

This logic of material disintegration reaches its apotheosis in Edwin Chadwick's descriptions of Lancashire colliers, whose skin got so dirty that it ceased to be like skin at all. In an interview on sanitary habits, one worker described his dirtiness in distinctly sartorial terms:

> "How often do the drawers (those employed in drawing coals) wash their bodies?"—"None of the drawers ever wash their bodies. I never wash my body; I let my shirt rub the dirt off; my shirt will show that. I wash my neck and ears, and face, of course."
>
> "Do you think it usual for the young women (engaged in the colliery) to do the same as you do?"—"I do not think it is usual for the lasses to wash their bodies; my sisters never wash themselves, and seeing is believing; they wash their faces, necks, and ears."
>
> "When a collier is in full dress, he has white stockings, and very tall shirt necks, very stiffly starched, and ruffles?"—"That is very sure, sir; but they never wash their bodies underneath; I know that; and their legs and bodies are as black as your hat." (Chadwick 315)

In the drawer's mind, wearing clothes is as good as washing (dirt will rub off on white cloth) even as unwashed skin is itself a form of clothing—in an odd transposition of anatomy and apparel, the collier's legs and body become the black hat that sets off the white stockings, collar, and ruffles of his formal attire. Allowing themselves to be permanently coated by coal, colliers regarded dirt almost as a garment, a protective barrier between the skin and the elements: one laborer claimed that being made to wash was "equal to robbing him of a great coat which he had had for some years" (quoted in Chadwick 316). Blurring the boundary between the skin and its coverings, blotting out

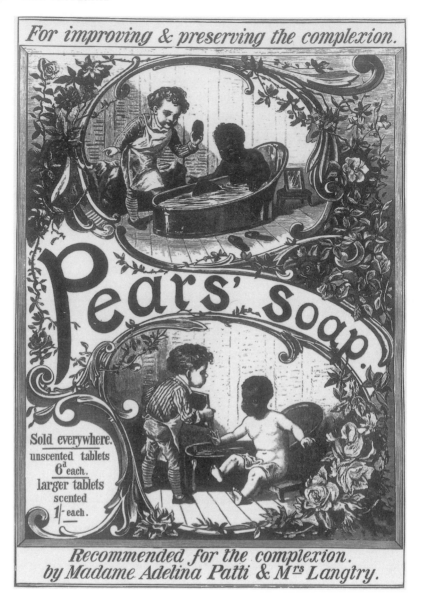

Fig. 5. Late-century advertisement for ethnic cleanser.

the line that divides the body from its belongings, the sheer intensity of the skin's pigment takes on the aspect of an overdyed item of outerwear, an old greatcoat or a gentleman's black hat. At once a valued possession and a social stigma, a manufactured covering and a degenerative coloring, black skin made bodies lose their distinctness *as* bodies, blending them into new material forms. The rhetoric of industrial dirt thus depicted blackness as a by-product of industry, a disposable commodity that could be worn, and even washed off: one advertisement for Pears' soap depicted bathing as a form of ethnic cleansing (fig. 5).

The discourse of cholera added a crucial dimension to this broad logic of blackening manufacture, depicting the disease as a pathological process that racialized its victims by converting them to dark raw materials. To be sick with Asiatic cholera, the literature suggested, was to be reduced to the raw materials of race; it was to have your body made into blackness itself. Although the means by which cholera was communicated from one person to the next was hotly debated, the metaphors used to describe the physical effects of the disease were surprisingly consistent across these debates, combining to develop an entire metaphorics of material conversion. Dramatically reproducing the chemical reactions of racial production, the bodies of cholera victims became a means of consolidating the essential—if essentially indeterminate—relationship between race and raw material in modern English society. Reducing the blood to its mineral constituents, cholera licensed a series of slippages among dark people and things, substances and skin: simply put, the choleraic body resembles a black person because it has dark things inside.

At points this epistemological endeavor centered on the deep blueness of cholera patients, likening their cyanotic skin to various industrial dyes and dips. As if coloring could kill, one account effectively suggested that death was due to dyeing: one corpse was blue "as if dip't in a solution of indigo" (quoted in Richardson 227); another was a victim of imperfect rinsing: like a badly laundered load, it bore the signs of having been "rubbed with a washerwoman's blue rag" (quoted in Longmate 88). More commonly, however, metaphors of choleraic materiality centered on blackness. "Black blood" was continually compared to black stuff: to tar (on bleeding, one woman's arm yielded "a few drops of tar-like blood" [Jameson 42]); to treacle (one sludgy vein yielded only a "trickling of dark treacly matter" [G. Johnson 24]); to ink (the gallbladder of one woman was "filled with acrid bile of inky blackness" [Jameson 50], while another corpse resembled a splattered clerk: "His nails look as if they had been stained with ink" [quoted in Longmate 88]); and even to coal (cholera "exerts the art of the collier, and fills your veins with charcoal" [Jameson 277]). Bringing the rhetoric of industrial dirt full circle, the coal in the veins of the cholera victim seemed to blacken his body into the form of a collier. Among other things, cholera mimicked the dustiness of industrial labor, making the victim's body seem to have been blackened by raw material: "In cases that terminate fatally, we find a peculiar dusky look, less bluish than heart cases, in fact really blackish. This is especially noticeable about the extremities. The appearance of the hands and feet may remind us of gangrene, but yet it differs in that there is a shriveled, shrunken look, and no purpling, the flesh tints showing as through coal dust" (Benson 99). Like Lamb's boyish sweep, whose rosy cheeks bloom through a new layer of soot, this account envisions the cholera victim as a grubby worker, a moribund miner whose fatal flaw is his failure to wash the coal dust from his hands and feet. The blood of cholera victims was thus seen as a chemical analogue of material culture. A sticky residue whose likeness was to be found both at home and in the street, it was a substance that could be all sorts of dark things at once.

Exotically dark and darkly indistinct, choleraic blood had a peculiarly ornamental effect. Autopsy reports developed an entire morbid aesthetics in attempting to capture its special character. One physician compared it to polished metal: "Looking at the blood in the bottom of a tin pan, it very much resembled a piece of metal which had been japanned black—it was highly polished, and looked as if the surface was covered with a pellicle; and in attempting to touch it with the finger, one had the impression that the surface would give resistance" (Jameson 142). Another saw choleraic blood as polish itself: "The blood of those attacked by cholera is so thick, that it will not flow from the vessels; its consistence is viscid, and very analogous to that of varnish" (Tardieu 39). (This particular physician described the entire corpse as a finished interior: in addition to the blood, "the peritoneal surface is, in all cases, sticky and shining as if varnished"; while the brain "is coated with a sort of sticky varnish" [Tardieu 33, 41]). Whether the blood was likened to treacle or tar; ink, lead, bronze, or coal; whether it was seen as varnished, polished, or japanned; the end result was the same—doctors envisioned the victim as a sort of shrink-wrapped corpse, a small quantity of black material packaged in paper (the classic choleraic tongue was "covered with a white slimy coat as thick as a sheet of paper" [quoted in Coventry 58]) and string (empty jugular veins had the "appearance of string[s] of twine," while drained arteries became rubber bands, "white-reddish shining cord[s], possessed of elasticity" [Jameson 56, 58]). Cholera thus wrapped up a substantive speciation that had been happening to the poor all along. Conjuring images of the dark side of English life, the disease was a pathological testament to the ease with which a body could be variously wrung out and sucked dry, wizened, wasted, and worn away by its encounter with a devastatingly modern world.

CRITICAL CONTAMINATION

Asiatic cholera died out in England in 1866, but its symbolic legacy lives on. We can see conceptual descendants of the cholera story in everything from Bram Stoker's *Dracula* (1897) (which also features an Eastern invader who remakes the English over in his own image by draining them dry) to AIDS, another exotic disease that has attacked the West in what many consider to be its weak spot (the difference is that the gay man has replaced the poor one as the infectious point of entry). We can also see this legacy in late-nineteenth- and early-twentieth-century nationalist discourse, which diagnoses both marginal ethnicities and pernicious state practices as forms of the Victorian disease: the protofascist German nationalism of the 1890s called the Jews a cholera, for example, while Trotsky called Stalinism a cholera (Sontag 82–83).[32] Finally, it is there in twentieth-century fiction: Thomas Mann's 1911 novella about an aging writer's morbid attraction to a young boy, *Death in Venice*, takes place during an outbreak of Asiatic cholera; Gabriel García Márquez's *Love in the Time of Cholera* (1985) follows suit, treating emotion as something whose contours are shaped by the particular exigencies of the disease.

More to the point, we can see something very like the rhetoric of cholera in postcolonial theory itself, which relies heavily on a vocabulary of contagion to describe the imperial imagination. Sometimes the presence of infection is fairly subtle, as when Benedict Anderson describes nationalism as something that "spreads."[33] At other times it is explicit, as when Simon During defines postcolonialism as "the need, in nations or groups which have been victims of imperialism, to achieve an identity uncontaminated by universalist or Eurocentric images" (125). Like any effective contamination, this one spreads into other texts, where it becomes a formative figure in their own critiques of empire. Building on During's argument, Linda Hutcheon argues that "the entire post-colonial project usually posits . . . the impossibility of [colonial] identity ever being 'uncontaminated'; just as the *word* post-colonialism holds within it its own 'contamination' by colonialism, so too does the culture itself" (171). And, building on Hutcheon, Diana Brydon argues that the contaminations of colonialism need not result in complicity—that "cultural contamination" might instead operate as a point of resistance for the colonized (191).[34] These are not isolated cases, but evidence of an analytical framework that is riddled with disease. In Edward Said's *Culture and Imperialism* (1993), for example, the problem is systemic. Noting that critics have historically tended to "sanitize" national culture "as a realm of unchanging intellectual monuments, free from worldly affiliations" (13), Said argues that the particular "challenge" facing criticism today is "*not* to see culture in this way— that is, as antiseptically quarantined from its worldly affiliations" (xiv). As if these opening images of infection were themselves infectious, the rest of Said's book is tinged with recurring references to the "infection," "infiltration," and "impurity" that is "symptomatic" of cultural formation under imperialism (for representative examples, see pp. 15, 68, 114, 188, 206, 210).[35] Taken together, these examples describe a sort of metaphorical infestation, a contagious language of contagion that makes what should be a theoretical problem—the historical role of the idea of contagion in the framing of global relations—into a strategy for theorizing those relations. As such, they show how contemporary critical discourse relies on a symbolic association between empire and disease very like that which animates Victorian writing about cholera. If, in cholera, we see an exotic contagion metaphorized as a form of colonial-ism, contemporary theories of colonialism frequently do just the re-verse, using contamination as a trope for the colonial encounter.

Of course, the imagery of contagion and disease circulates freely in contemporary criticism, where it provides a sort of all-purpose figure for cultural, authorial, and textual influences. But those metaphors take on a particularly troubling cast when they appear in writing that is attempting to historicize—and even to change—global distributions of power. Read alongside the history of cholera, the examples cited above highlight how a central metaphoric formation of postcolonial critical language is embedded in the ideological patterns it seeks to uncover and resist. For it is not simply that postcolonial discourse has internalized a rhetoric of contamination, but rather that it uses that rhetoric critically, as a way to describe the phenomenon of cultural contamination. This is catachresis in action—so thoroughly has contamination infiltrated postcolonial thought that we have no other language for the thing it describes. (At the end of *Culture and Imperialism,* Said admits this: "Contamination is the wrong word to use," he writes; "but some notion of literature and indeed all culture as hybrid [in Homi Bhabha's com-plex sense of that word] and encumbered, or entangled and overlapping with what used to be regarded as extraneous elements—this strikes me as *the* essential idea for the revolutionary realities today" [317].) The price of such structuring motifs should be clear in light of this chapter: for the critical fascination with contagion as a figure for the colonial encounter has gone hand in hand with a failure to appreciate how real diseases such as cholera have helped to structure the imperial imagina-tion (an imagination that in turn inevitably informs its own critique).[36] The result is symptomatic (there is no other word for it) of the problem, a criticism whose capacity for radically rewriting history is diminished in proportion to the degree that its language contains the traces of rhetorical patterns whose ideological valences it has itself forgotten.

That the language of postcolonial critique may at points do more to repress memory than revive it is perhaps best seen in Said's discussion of *Death in Venice,* which reads the story as a parable for how an awareness of empire materially affected modernist aesthetics even as it fails to notice the very material dimensions of Mann's disease metaphors: "In

Mann's great fable of the alliance between creativity and disease . . . the plague that infects Europe is Asiatic in origin; the combination of dread and promise, of degeneration and desire, so effectively rendered by Aschenbach's psychology is Mann's way of suggesting . . . that Europe, its art, mind, monuments, is no longer invulnerable, no longer able to ignore its ties to its overseas domains" (*Culture and Imperialism* 188). For Said, Mann's Asiatic "plague" exists purely as a textual trope, a way of indicating a historically specific dilemma of cultural formation. What this reading misses, though, is precisely what Said's entire study is committed to discovering: the historical context that enabled such a trope to take shape in the first place. As we have seen, Asiatic cholera can fuel a parable about cultural mixing because it had, by 1911, already taken shape *as* a parable for cultural mixing. When Mann invokes Asiatic cholera, he does so in a climate that understands the disease not as a colorful version of that larger, vaguely literary category, "plague," but as itself.

What is lost in Said's account is how much Mann's exotic modernism owes to nineteenth-century ideas about cholera. Mann narrates the disease just as Victorian doctors did, noting its source in "the hot, moist swamps of the delta of the Ganges, where it bred in the mephitic air of that primeval island-jungle"; tracking its "spread" from Hindustan (where it "rage[s] with great violence") to China, Persia, and Moscow "while Europe trembled lest the spectre be seen striding westward"; and noting its arrival in Italy in the form of two "emaciated, blackened corpses." He describes the disease itself in classically medical terms: "Recoveries were rare. Eighty out of every hundred died, and horribly, for the onslaught was of the extremest violence, and not infrequently of the 'dry' type, the most malignant form of the contagion. In this form the victim's body loses power to expel the water secreted by the blood-vessels, it shrivels up, he passes with hoarse cries from convulsion to convulsion, his blood grows thick like pitch, and he suffocates in a few hours" (63–64). The clinical accuracy of Mann's depiction of cholera is itself part of the story's motor, the materialization of the metaphoric dis-ease that sends Aschenbach to Venice in the first place. Walking one evening in Munich, Aschenbach is attacked by a spiritual analogue of the cholera that eventually kills him: like an "unexpected contagion" (6), the "longing to travel" not only hits him with the characteristic

violence of cholera ("such suddenness and passion as to resemble a sei-
zure") but also causes a "hallucination" that "projected" his "desire" as
that which is born out of the same fecund conditions that foster cholera:

> He beheld a landscape, a tropical marshland, beneath a reeking sky,
> steaming, monstrous, rank—a kind of primeval wilderness-world of
> islands, morasses, and alluvial channels. Hairy palm-trunks rose
> near and far out of lush brakes of fern, out of bottoms of crass
> vegetation, fat, swollen, thick with incredible bloom. There were
> trees, mis-shapen as a dream, that dropped their naked roots straight
> through the air into the ground or into water that was stagnant and
> shadowy and glassy-green, where mammoth milk-white blossoms
> floated, and strange high-shouldered birds with curious bills stood
> gazing sidewise without sound or stir. Among the knotted joints of a
> bamboo thicket the eyes of a crouching tiger gleamed—and he felt
> his heart throb with terror, yet with a longing inexplicable. Then the
> vision vanished. (5-6)

If Aschenbach's world-weariness manifests itself as a positively choleric
fantasy of change, his death by cholera must be read as a dream come a
little bit too true. The richness of Mann's handling of modernist malaise thus depends on the specificity of Asiatic cholera as a set of symptoms that are always also a set of signs—a specificity his audience would
have known as well as he.[37] In Said's reading of Mann's story, however,
Asiatic cholera is so entirely subsumed within an untheorized rhetoric
of contagion that its own historical status as a very real source of both
exotic infection and imperial figuration is completely lost. The disease
is not even properly named.

Cultural systems being what they are, we cannot say that postcolonial theory is *about* cholera—it would be a real stretch to argue that
Asiatic cholera has directly affected or determined the self-consciously
radical vocabulary employed by contemporary critiques of imperialism.
But if Said's undiagnosed case of cholera proves anything, it is that
the two discourses have enough in common that they demand to be
thought together, especially since they occupy such radically different
political and historical positions. Thinking the connection between
cholera—a Victorian disease that originally supplied the means of
framing a protonationalist rhetoric of racial threat—and postcolonial

thought—a radical late-twentieth-century interrogation of modern Western notions of race and nation—would mean, first of all, asking what this forgotten moment of Orientalist imagining might be able to tell us about the peculiar power of imperialist rhetorical systems. And it would mean asking whether, and to what extent, our techniques for interrogating those systems end up reproducing them.

Such an analysis would begin by observing that the continuities between postcolonial theory and Asiatic cholera extend beyond metaphor to method. For long before postcolonial criticism hit on the idea of cultural contamination, Asiatic cholera had been used as a strategy of critique. As I noted earlier, Asiatic cholera lies at the heart of one of the first sustained critiques of modern Western industrial culture— something the Victorians themselves were quick to point out. Pinpointing the most wretched rookeries and squalid dens with scary regularity, Asiatic cholera was metaphorized as a microscopic muckraker, a germinal snoop with an instinctual ability to uncover the most degraded pockets of metropolitan space. To take just two examples: in 1849, the *Edinburgh Review* called cholera a "health inspector, who . . . points out with terrible distinctness and unfailing accuracy those districts which are not only occasionally the regions of death, but at all times the nurseries of disease" ("Supply of Water to the Metropolis" 389). Likewise, in 1848 the *London Times* called cholera "the best of all sanitary reformers," an unrelenting expository force that "overlooks no mistake, and pardons no oversight" (quoted in Wohl 117; Bynum 55). So it was that the symbolic linking of race and contagion that we see in Asiatic cholera ultimately fueled a progressive politics of urban renewal. The story of an Eastern invader who enters white working-class bodies and then turns them black motivated a series of necessary social reforms in ways more deadly but more commonplace diseases such as typhus, tuberculosis, and influenza never could. Cleaner and more plentiful water for drinking, washing, and cooking; regular trash removal; better sewerage; stricter housing codes; and more sanitary burial practices were but a few of the positive results to come from cholera's inflammatory rhetoric of colonization and racial conversion.

Asiatic cholera was thus both a form of cultural imperialism and an important technique of social criticism; it was, indeed, cultural imperialism *as* social criticism, an infectious logic of national and corporeal threat that became the basis of the new social science that eventually evolved into modern sociology. In this context, we need to see Asiatic cholera as more than just an intriguing moment in the history of empire, a scene of Orientalist imagining that tells us a great deal about how Victorians conflated questions of race, disease, and economic growth. We also need to regard Asiatic cholera as an important moment in the history of the history of imperialism, a signal moment of national self-imagining whose symbolic strategies filter through our own formulations as a series of highly curious rhetorical effects. If postcolonial theory uses a language of contamination and spread to describe imperialist patterns of conceptual violence, that is because it has caught that language from its historical antecedents—as Said himself puts it, "there is no just way in which the past can be quarantined from the present" (4).[38] And as such it forcibly performs the need for a scholarship that can accommodate the inevitable impurity of any critical endeavor. For if the example of postcolonial theory can tell us anything, it is that it is the nature of even the most self-consciously revisionary criticism to seep into, and be infected by, the thing it studies. The symptomatic integrity of Said's dictum—as tainted as it is true—may thus be said to diagnose the critical condition of this book, whose efforts to track linguistic and conceptual continuities between Victorian models of illness (often also models of culture) and contemporary models of culture (always also carriers of culture) mark its own strategic impurity, its desire to embody a historiography that figures its own distortions into the past it seeks to shape.

TWO

Breast Reductions

This chapter begins with the history of a word. Since at least the sixteenth century, an income has been an almost exclusively economic entity: a payment, a revenue, interest. From the fourteenth to the eighteenth centuries, an ancome was a morbid entity: a swelling, a tumor, a growth. A funny thing happened around 1800: the word *ancome* disappeared, and people began calling bodily tumors and growths *incomes*. The first recorded instance of this was in 1808, when one dictionary defined *income* as "a morbid affection of any part of the body, a swelling, impostume, tumour, or the like." In the early years of the nineteenth century, incomes suddenly became grotesque hybrids, part money and part pathology—a means of livelihood and a potentially life-threatening condition.[1] In this hybrid guise incomes began to appear in medical literature, novels, and stories. In 1858, for instance, one of these mixed incomes appeared in a strange little tale entitled *Rab and His Friends*. Written by the Scottish physician John Brown, the story is itself a weird hybrid—half sentimental animal tale (Rab is a dog), half medical memoir (Rab's mistress, Ailie, has breast cancer). Early in the story, Ailie's husband describes her delicate symptoms to the doctor: "She's got a trouble in her breest," he says; "some kind o' an income, we're thinkin'" (13). The narrative that follows is based closely on a case Brown himself saw treated in Edinburgh, and its centerpiece is a detailed account of

Ailie's mastectomy, which is performed before a theater of medical students. The medical students weep as they watch the unanesthetized operation, but the patient is absolutely silent and still. When it is over, she stands, bows to the audience, says that she hopes she has not behaved ill, and walks out. A few days later, Ailie dies from infection, deliriously singing fragments of lullabies as she holds a pillow to her missing breast, nursing it like a baby. Then her husband dies of grief. And then the dog dies of grief. The End.[2]

It is a creepy, sad story, not least because it is a tale whose sentimentalism hinges on a failure of sense. The notion of a malignant "income" in the breast conjures a series of nonsensical associations, seems somehow to align getting sick with getting paid: as if cancer were a kind of internal revenue, and tumors were somehow peculiarly "economic" growths. The word *income* is, indeed, a kind of false figure, an allusion to nowhere, a metaphor that it makes no sense to read; and as such it points to the special linguistic and conceptual problem posed by breast cancer during the nineteenth century. For incomes are only part of the diseased breast's confused economy, whose clinical signs include all the elements of the modern industrial city—mass production, overcrowding, unsanitary environments, and, of course, prostitution. Indeed, so strong are the linguistic associations between breast cancer and urban culture that the disease appears insensibly, nonsensically, to follow a distinctly urban pattern of decay. Even so, these parallels are, like Ailie's income, peculiarly abortive. Just as *income* conjures an economic association it cannot sustain (cancers are hardly payoffs), so the discourse of breast cancer cuts short its own economic allusions. Employing the principal figures of Victorian political economy without any apparent awareness of political economy as such, the discourse of breast cancer forges its modern scientific identity by, paradoxically, making analogies that it does not make.[3] Reproducing a vocabulary from elsewhere—a vocabulary that it neither acknowledges nor appears to know—the discourse of breast cancer uses connotation denotatively, as the raw material of a neutral language of objective description.

That language is my subject here. This chapter concentrates on the discourse of breast cancer as it manifested itself between the 1850s, when cell theory revolutionized thinking about cancer, and the 1890s, when the radical mastectomy became the first viable treatment for the disease. These years mark a time of profound disjunction between medical theory and clinical practice, of unprecedented advancement in the conceptualization of cancer but relatively little change in the actual management of the disease. Though treatments ranging from surgery to compression to the application of caustics had been tried for hundreds of years, most doctors agreed that treatment had little, if any, positive effect; many felt that it only made things worse (Ailie's fatal mastectomy is a case in point). Indeed, as late as midcentury, doctors were debating whether breast cancer ought to be treated at all. During the second half of the nineteenth century, breast cancer became something to watch and study, and medical discussion of the subject centered more on etiological issues—what caused it, how it spread, what it *was*— than on treatment. As a consequence, Victorian writing on breast cancer is largely descriptive, committed, for lack of either etiologic or therapeutic certainty, to telling us what cancer is like: describing how it presents itself to the patient; how it reveals itself to hand and eye; how its cells look under the microscope; how it starts, spreads, recurs, and kills.

During these years, cancer operated as an ontological problem: if it could not yet be reliably treated, it was at least something that physicians were newly equipped to understand. Mid- to late-century writing about cancer consequently represents a systematic effort not only to render cancer recognizable in all its phases, to distinguish it from benign growths and to differentiate among its varied forms, but also to find a properly scientific language for the disease itself. The language that emerged was a mélange of vocabularies, inconsistent on the level of theory as well as on the level of diction. Though cell theory radically transformed thinking about cancer, it did not wholly displace existing ideas about cancer's origins (that it began in the blood or the nerves, or that it was the result of some kind of contagion); nor did it completely supplant the often figural, suggestive vocabularies associated with these theories.[4] To read nineteenth-century writing on cancer—breast cancer in particular—is thus to encounter a strange linguistic mixture, a hodgepodge of vocabularies traceable to such disparate and discontinuous roots as an obsolete humoral theory, eighteenth-century pathophysiology, a nascent psychology, modern cell theory, and—strangely enough— Victorian political economy.

It is intuitively obvious why the discourse of breast cancer would contain so many competing medical voices—change is gradual, and languages, like bodies, always contain vestigial structures, signs of an older, increasingly inoperative mode of being. It is less obvious why that discourse would import a distinctly sociological rhetoric to describe the physiology of metastatic disease, particularly given medicine's growing emphasis on the importance of working within neutral, nonmetaphorical language. But that is just what happened. At precisely the moment that Victorian social critics were beginning to give particular attention to that quintessentially modern formation, the industrial city, the language of breast cancer began to be filled with the very words and phrases that were being used to describe the special problems arising from England's massive, rapid, and deeply troubling economic growth. This chapter focuses on this bizarre convergence, tracking a series of striking correspondences between the newly modernized discourse of breast cancer and an emergent discourse on modernization. My aim is both historical and methodological: to examine how the massive cultural shifts entailed by urbanization inflected medical understanding of breast cancer, and to examine the terms on which we license ourselves to make such historical assessments in the first place.[5]

On first glance, the presence of cultural criticism in medical writing about breast cancer looks like a simple case of social commentary. Describing breast disease in terms of the stock categories of urban-industrial description—commodities, crowds, slums—medicine appears to be using cancer to conduct a coded examination of modern gender norms: What, medicine seems to ask, is the effect of growth on gender? More generally, what is the status of gender in an era of growth? On second glance, however, the relationship between these two discourses proves to be far more complex. Like Ailie's fixed income, medicine's economic allusions frustrate the questions they seem to invite. Breast cancer's metaphors are analogical—and analytical—dead ends, situated so as to cut short, rather than encourage, their own connotations. Full of figures that aren't images, Victorian writing about breast cancer poses a peculiar problem for cultural analysis, whose defining project is, to say the least, ill prepared to tackle breast cancer's most provocative suggestion: that the suggestive language of breast cancer ought not to be read as such. In order to address the historical and methodological complexities of Victorian writing about breast cancer, I have adopted a distinctly unorthodox writing strategy. This chapter takes shape as two adjacent entities, a pair of separate but symmetrical units whose respective contents are at once entirely incompatible with and utterly essential to each other. The first treats breast cancer's metaphors *as* metaphors, reading the diseased breast's "urbanity" as a coded commentary on the place of femininity in machine culture. The second uncovers the analytical premises of the first. Analyzing the sheer pathology of what may initially seem to be a perfectly sound cultural analysis, this section revisits questions of context and inflection in order to consider the possibility that these metaphors do not work metaphorically. Structured as a theoretical double take, this chapter argues that breast cancer has more to tell us about our own techniques for thinking culture than it does about Victorian models of gender per se. And it locates that lesson not in contemporary debates about method, but in the discourse of breast cancer itself. For far from enacting a metaphoric commentary on its own historical moment, breast cancer's cultural metaphors turn out to frame a set of pressing questions about the nature of cultural commentary itself.

DIAGNOSIS

Victorian physicians understood cancer as a disease of modernity. More common in industrialized countries than in undeveloped ones, physicians argued that cancer was a function of "civilization," a by-product or side effect of progress. In his 1885 inquiry into the causes of cancer Willard Parker writes: "We shall be obliged to look for causes which exist in civilized communities, and which are absent, or almost entirely absent, among barbarous or uncivilized communities, or among nations whose modes of life are essentially different from ours. For—and this is an extremely significant circumstance,—it has been found that barbarous and semi-civilized peoples are comparatively free—some tribes, indeed, are perfectly free—from cancer. Then again we shall find communities among civilized nations who have certain peculiar habits, which somewhat resemble those of natural or rude peoples, who have very little cancer" (36–37). Cancer came with growth—one physician

wrote that cities often had "a malignant habit" (Banks 1138)—and as
such, it was a handy figure for modern social ills. Robert Southey, for
instance, saw capitalism as a malignant cultural development: "The
growth might have been checked, if the consequences had been apprehended in time; but now it has acquired so great a bulk, its nerves
have branched so widely, and the vessels of the tumour are so inoscu-
lated into some of the principal veins and arteries of the natural system,
that to remove it by absorption is impossible, and excision will be fatal"
(quoted in Ure 277–78). At once a material effect of modern industrial
culture and a metaphor for the material effects of that culture, cancer
developed a very realistic symbolic economy, one whose import was
significantly modulated by the modern economic state.

Breast cancer occupied a special place in this pathologic. Because
it affected women almost exclusively, it was a distinctly gendered form
of the civilized disease.[6] Said to be caused by just about everything
(Parker's book lists "age, marriage or celibacy, menstruation, lacta-
tion, depraved habits, mental affliction, sustained intellectual labor,
social condition, climate, and geographical location" as contributing
factors [40]), breast cancer seemed to be brought about by the simple
fact of being female in a rapidly changing world. Such an expansive
etiology had far-reaching symbolic implications. As a side effect of
"civilization" that killed women, breast cancer implicitly embodied the
possibility that modernization was inherently hostile to female nature;
in other words, it raised the possibility that women could die from
development. That suggestion is carried through the discourse of breast
cancer, which imports the language of growing economies into the
densely feminine space of the breast in such a way as to suggest that it is
not simply women who die of development, but the idea of Woman
itself.

In order to see how this may be so, we must begin by tracing the
semantic contours of the breast. Breasts carried a great deal of symbolic weight in Victorian culture. Since the eighteenth century they
had substantiated essentialist conceptions of gender, making palpable
the premise that women are meant to be wives and mothers. "Nature
destined this organ to nourish the new-born human being," one physician wrote, "she gave to the breast a seductive charm by virtue of its

form and bloom which powerfully attracts men; this is why jealous husbands and discreet wives, do not permit its charms to be paraded" (quoted in Jordanova 29).[7] As this quote suggests, the healthy breast literally supported social fictions about women's nature; indeed, as a metonymy for a woman's essential self, it was a symbolic structure in its own right.

The breast's figural dimensions are perhaps most clear in literary texts, where the breast—that classic metonymy for "heart"—stands as a repository of feeling and sources of emotional sustenance. Dickens's Florence Dombey, for instance, keeps "glowing love" (*Dombey and Son* 328), a "deep secret" (396), a "cruel wound" (397), a "load of sacred care" (424), "hope" (478), and "pity" (800) in her "overcharged and heavy-laden breast" (316); while Little Dorrit's "innocent breast," a "fountain of love and fidelity that never ran dry or waned," keeps her insolvent father in "a reasonable flow of spirits" (*Little Dorrit* 274). Mrs. Micawber's miraculous ability to produce milk performs a similar function, feeding her babies and also buoying her husband's unsinkable optimism: the Micawbers might have a cash flow problem, but "Nature's founts," Micawber gushes, never run dry (*David Copperfield* 315). Proper women edit themselves, preventing unhealthy feelings from growing inside them by killing off emotional excess (in George Meredith's *The Egoist* Laetitia Dale dutifully stifles her unrequited love for Sir Willoughby by giving "a wrench to the neck of the young hope in her breast" [32]). By contrast, women who give their feelings too much sway are morally compromised (in *Little Dorrit*, Miss Wade suffers the "miseries of a morbid breast" [727]). Still others are emotionally underdeveloped. The size of Mrs. Merdle's breasts indicates the depth of her insensitivity—she needs "room enough to be unfeeling in" (*Little Dorrit* 287)—and the second Mrs. Dombey is simply hollow inside: "'Never seek to find in me,'" she says, "laying her hand upon her breast, 'what is not here.' . . . 'The germ of all that purifies a woman's breast, and makes it true and good, has never stirred in mine'" (*Dombey and Son* 590, 474). The textualization of female flesh in Victorian novels is so complete that the breast shapes the contours of the self it symbolizes: well-rounded women simply overflow with good feeling while lesser figures suffer from a sort of emotional deficit—they have either mood swings or a flat affect.

Medicine not only participated in this literary shorthand, it also solidified the symbolic content of the breast into scientific fact by assigning the healthy breast an emotional anatomy—its physiology *was* its deep capacity for feeling. Such "close sympathies exist between the ovaries and breasts" (Birkett 16) that the development of the breasts at puberty takes place as an act of anatomical solidarity: as if to make a strong show of support, "the whole organ, sympathizing with ovarian development, becomes completely changed, and that which previously was simply rudimentary, becomes fitted to perform the functions for which it has been provided by nature—the nourishment of the future offspring" (Birkett 2). So strong is this organic affinity that breasts are acutely distressed by menopause—"The final stoppage of the menstruation is known to produce certain 'sympathetic' movements in the breasts; they sometimes even enlarge and discharge a milky secretion" (Creighton, *Contributions* 176). Situated at the center of a woman's being, the breast stands as a profoundly womanly entity, one whose day-to-day existence is defined by the tender palpitations of a sensitive soul, and whose rational behavior comes only irregularly, in spurts ("Woman's reason," writes George Meredith, "is in the milk of her breasts" [*Ordeal of Richard Feverel* 444]). Merging mammary function with a normative idea of gender, medicine formulated a literary biology, a metaphoric materiality in which breast and text merge into a physically grounded fiction of femininity: in Victorian medicine, the breast is a little woman in its own right.

As such, the breast became a principal point of reference in Victorian social theory, which held it up as a sign of women's natural and necessary separateness from public, industrial space. According to both conservative and radical commentators, factory work prevented women from learning decent values and domestic habits (female factory workers supposedly made bad wives, careless mothers, and turned all too readily to prostitution). It also kept their bodies, particularly their breasts, from developing properly (a working woman couldn't be a good mother even if she wanted to).[8] Drawing on its power as a symbol of women's reproductive destiny, reformers fixed on the slack, wasted breasts of working women as a tangible image of tapped-out sexuality. In *Artisans and Machinery* (1836), for example, Peter Gaskell writes that factory labor masculinizes women, clinching his argument by contending that machine work saps breasts of their natural vitality: "Very early in life, from ten to fourteen years, the breasts [of factory girls] are often found large and firm, and highly sensitive, whilst at a later period—at a period indeed when they should show the greatest activity and vital energy—when in fact they have children to support from them, they are soft, flaccid, and pendulous, and very unirritable—both states giving the most decisive proofs of perversion in the usual functional adaptation of parts" (189). Where Gaskell believed that factories drained the female body of its reproductive power, Engels worried that women's maternal nature was spilling over into industrial space. In *The Condition of the Working Class in England* (1845), he characterizes the factory as an inhospitable receptacle of mother's milk: " 'M.H., twenty years old, has two children, the youngest a baby, that is tended by the other, a little older. The mother goes to the mill shortly after five o'clock in the morning, and comes home at eight at night; all day the milk pours from her breasts, so that her clothing drips with it.' 'H.W. has three children, goes away Monday morning at five o'clock, and comes back Saturday evening; has so much to do for the children then that she cannot get to bed before three o'clock in the morning; often wet through to the skin, and obliged to work in that state.' She said: 'My breasts have given me the most frightful pain, and I have been dripping wet with milk' " (153). Citing the testimony of women whose breasts overflowed on the job, Engels uses the leaky gland as a trope for the dissolution of working-class values: "The employment of the wife dissolves the family utterly and of necessity" (153). Breasts thus enable both Gaskell and Engels to assert that female bodies and machines are inherently antithetical structures. Dripping where they shouldn't and drooping before their time, they are anatomical evidence that maternal instincts and modern industry cannot come together without harming one or the other, or both (Engels implies that female factory labor is not only bad for the family but is also hard on the machines).[9]

It is in this context that we can begin to trace the significance of medical writing about breast cancer. Just as women laborers compromised their femininity (a compromise that was felt most painfully in their alternately underdeveloped or overblown breasts), so cancerous breasts went bad by going to work. Characterized by the rapid and uncontrolled proliferation of cells, cancer was commonly blamed on what doctors routinely called "excessive production" (Creighton, *Contributions* 37), a fatal manufacture of cells which, they said, serves "*no useful purpose and tend[s] to persist and increase without respect to those influences by which the organic economy is maintained*" (Deaver and McFarland 331; original emphasis). Remarkable for what Sir James Paget calls its "inherent power of self-maintenance" (*Surgical Pathology* 702), the cancerous breast is depicted as a self-operating system whose yield is dangerously in "excess of normal development and growth" (Gross 1), and whose ill effects stem from its "surplus vitality" (Parker 58). The malignant mass is a mass production in its own right, manufacturing so many cells that they eventually pile up in the heaps of waste material we know as tumors.

Just as factory labor was felt to destroy a woman's moral fiber, leading her away from duty toward a life of drink, dissipation, and even prostitution, so too did the diseased breast exhibit the telltale signs of degeneration. Breast cancer embodies a sort of moral-material failure, a process in which both feelings and the flesh that contains them break down. Marked by a "decline in the integrity of the breast tissues" (Deaver and McFarland 477), cancerous flesh undergoes a kind of nervous breakdown: cancer is a "disorder of function" (Creighton, *Contributions* 177) that manifests itself as a functional disorder, a "diseased excitation" (Creighton, *Contributions* 174) in which the breast suffers from a loss of proper feeling.[10] Originating as an "affection" (Sheild 334) brought on by "exciting causes" (usually "irritation"), one whose symptoms are acutely feminine (the diseased breast "blushes," "dimples," and even "puckers up"), cancer embodies a dramatic change of "disposition" (Gross 6) in which "innocent" tissue becomes increasingly "bossy," "indolent," and "tense"; develops a tendency to "embarrass" (Nunn 14) nearby tissues; and finally "hardens" into a "degenerate" type.[11] If medicine understood the healthy breast as a synecdoche for femininity, a repository for the personal qualities that make a woman essentially herself, it held up the diseased one as a deviation from sociosexual norms.

Although medical books advised that "every *tumor be removed before it has time or opportunity to misbehave*" (Deaver and McFarland 334; original emphasis), this recommendation was more a disciplinary fantasy than a practical clinical rule. Many women did not visit the doctor until the disease was far advanced—disfiguring, even ulcerating. And surgical techniques were crude. Until the last few years of the nine-teenth century, more women died from breast surgery than were cured by it. Doctors cut on unanesthetized flesh with unsterile knives; they dug out diseased tissue with their fingers and staunched bleeding with acid and tar. In short, the reality was that once a growth got going, it was all but impossible to control it. In breast cancer, the flesh inevitably bore the brunt of the worry and stress that were associated with the onset of disease: it literally fell apart. Such a formulation makes perfect synecdochal sense—after all, the primary cause of breast cancer was, more often than not, the worry and stress associated with modern women's lives. Jut as excessive stress and suffering were said to bring about breast cancer, so too was the disease figured as a sort of material disturbance, a potentially life-threatening loss of fleshly equanimity.

Victorian social theory used the breast to signal a basic impasse between femininity and machinery; the breast could function as a regis-ter for debates about industrialism precisely because its essential differ-ence from public space was never in question. By contrast, the can-cerous breast appeared to do precisely the type of labor that many social critics felt was inherently hostile to women's sexuality. That labor was itself profoundly productive, transforming breast tissue so dramatically that it became virtually impossible to talk about it *as* breast tissue. Instead, doctors figured breast cancer as an elaborate material conver-sion, a pathological process of "mimicry" (Creighton, *Contributions* 180) in which the flesh makes itself over in the image of various physical forms.[12] Tumors are never simply tumors in breast cancer; they are always named after other things. Those things, moreover, are always the same; words used to describe tumors recur with mechanical regular-ity. Producing masses the size and consistency of "chestnuts" (Gross 57), "filberts" (17), "walnuts" (24), "nutmegs" (Birkett 91), "eggs" (Gross 24; Birkett 91), "butter," and even "cheese" (Velpeau 58), the cancerous breast converts simple flesh to an impressive, if sickening, bill of fare.[13] Automatically likening masses to the same old things over and over again, medical texts figure the cancerous breast as a sort of physiological food mill, a rapid stringing together of vegetable matter (on dissection, the "mammillary vein" of one woman was found to be "full of knots, which were cancerous, and hung much like a rope of onions" [quoted in Power 33]). While the bulk of tumors concentrate on quantity, turning out a quick succession of fairly basic forms (one mass changed from an English walnut to a bunch of peas to an orange to an egg before it was removed [Gross 150–51]), others are more exacting: one "lardaceous" cancer even cooked up a "brioche."[14] Manufacturing cells at a prodigious rate, the pathology of mass production makes up a gross anatomy of damaged goods—the cheeses are bad ("knotty . . . and ulcerated" [Velpeau 58]), the nutmegs are soft ("filled with reddish fluid" [Birkett 91]), and the eggs are of impossible dimensions (one "goose egg" achieved a length of twelve inches and a weight of seven pounds over a twelve-year period; another reached a circumference of twenty-two inches and weighed four pounds after twenty years [Gross 57]).[15] Of course, analogies between tumors and produce go back at least as far as Galen. Medical accounts of cancer have always compared the size, shape, and consistency of cancerous growths to various foods. In nineteenth-century accounts, though, this language takes on a new, distinctly modern aspect. Tied to a vocabulary of production, excess, and waste, the fruits of cancer appear less as "natural" growths than as the perverse products of an indiscriminate system of manufacture (one that not only does not know when to stop, but presumes to mass-produce things that cannot be "made"). Taking shape as the scene of productive excess, the sick breast figures as a physiological factory system run amok.

Flesh disappeared from the language of breast cancer at the moment of its own inscription; able to talk about it only metaphorically, medicine developed a symbolic machinery whose basic parameters formed a curious analogue to popular accounts of the nineteenth-century marketplace. Just as writing about breast cancer figured diseased flesh as that which has become something else, Victorian descriptions of urban space relied on a sort of squashed iconography, a language that conjured the crowded, noisy, smelly reality of the city by symbolically crushing disparate material forms into one another. This pattern of conflation is best seen in *London Labour and the London Poor* (1861), Henry Mayhew's massive mid-century study of urban street life. Describing the street markets as having "more of the character of a fair than a market" (1:9), Mayhew depicts the "scramble that is going on throughout London for a living" as a "riot" full of "confusion and uproar" (1:10), a carnivalesque environment in which people not only get jumbled with other people—"the boy's sharp cry, the woman's cracked voice, the gruff, hoarse shout of the man, are all mingled together" (1:9)—but also wind up inextricably entangled with things. Street sellers, for instance, are metonymically identified with what they sell, so that individual men come to be known as "pickled whelks" (1:158); "sweet-stuffs" (1:158), "baked taties" (1:174), "plum duffers" (1:198), and even "ham-sandwiches" (1:177). Moreover, Mayhew's representation of the city as a scene of fluid boundaries where such "ellipses, or abbreviations, are common" (1:158) assigns women sellers a particularly elemental relationship to goods—men costermongers are classified by commodities, but women sellers seem to turn into them. One old woman has a "little 'button' of a nose, with the nostrils entering her face like bullet holes" (1:110), while another "old dame" has "a face wrinkled like a dried plum" (1:110). The streets of London are jammed with these composite figures; Mayhew describes "six women, with baskets of dried herrings . . . crouching in a line on the kerbstone with the fish before them; their legs . . . drawn up so closely to their bodies that the shawl covered the entire figure and they looked very like the podgy 'tombolers' sold by the Italian boys" (1:109), and even observes a group of girls with "japanned" hair ("black . . . smoothed with grease, and shining" [1:110]). The mess and danger of modern urban life are thus exemplified most perfectly by the image of the woman who has blended into her surroundings so totally that she cannot be separated from the streets she walks and the things she sells. Variously varnished and stuffed and stitched together, crazy combinations of flesh and other materials, the women vendors come to embody the characteristics of commodities themselves. One woman even "sat, literally packed in a sort of hamper-basket" alongside her fruit stall, like a particularly fragile piece of produce (1:463).

Although female bodies are continually turning into commodities in Mayhew's sociology, these elisions are finally more a rhetorical device than real description, a means of indicating the sheer physical stress of life in the streets. Mayhew's metaphors signal the objectifying power of poverty, the reduction of the self to mere mechanical existence—the coster-girl's "mind, heart, soul are all absorbed in the belly" and she becomes a "locomotive stomach" (1:46). In so doing, these images humanize their subjects, showing them to be worth more than the things to which they are compared. By contrast, the descriptive language of cancer disintegrates the difference between female body and external object so completely that the two cannot be told apart. When cancer's figures echo those of material culture, they operate to erase not only a sense of self, but also a sense of flesh. Breast cancer describes a very real conversion—so real, in fact, that at points the new material realizes its own metaphoric construction. "Cheesy" tumors, for example, were well known to contain real cheese, the curdled products of diseased milk ducts.[16]

As the parallels between medicine and Mayhew's descriptions of the working poor indicate, breast cancer's "progress" forms a sort of linguistic analogue to the deeply critical accounts of social progress generated by Victorian reformers. In the new sociology, mass production leads to overcrowding, which in turn leads to the potential for mass violence and epidemic disease. This is as true for radicals such as Marx and Engels as it is for more conservative thinkers such as Mayhew and Chadwick. It is also the pattern of breast cancer, whose downward spiral reads like an embodied version of the story social critics were telling about a new, specifically modern form of social decay. Indeed, breast cancer echoes the words and figures of Victorian social criticism so faithfully that at times it is difficult to tell them apart. Some examples: Marx and others refer to the working classes as an "indefinite, disintegrated mass."[17] "Disintegrated mass" (Erichsen 695) is also a recurring phrase for the heterogeneous, decomposing tumor. And like Marx's "indefinite, disintegrated mass," the "disintegrated masses" of cancer comprise a sort of lumpenproletariat in their own right, an unstable grouping of cells whose tremendous energy absolutely threatens the stability of the system. Healthy bodies, Virchow famously observed, are like well-run states.[18] Cancer, by contrast, represents a visceral uprising, a loss of equanimity caused by the violence of unruly masses. Remarkable for the "disorderly crowding of their elements" (Paget, *Surgical Pathology* 691), tumors in the breast are violent combinations; "irritable" and "intolerant of manipulation" (Gross 60), they make up a disordered, disorderly threat to a healthy bodily order. Breast cancer's masses form a sort of molecular mob that destroys everything in its path—the "chief characteristic" of cancer, writes Paget, is its "invasion of all tissues, as if indifferently" (*Surgical Pathology* 696).[19] The French theorist Gustave Le Bon writes that crowds are distinguished by "the purely destructive nature of their power" (xviii). Cancers in turn behave like crowds in their tendency to "gradually and slowly advance, often uncontrolled and apparently uncontrollable, until death terminates the sufferings of the patient" (Birkett 227). Cancer thus realizes a revolutionary teleology in which the "spontaneity and self-governing properties of the cell" (Creighton, *Contributions* 5) are replaced by a widespread movement to overthrow the system as a whole (masses use force when they have to: one pushed its way out of the breast with "one-third of a fist" [Gross 52]). Overcrowding, it seems, is as common in the unregulated economies of cancerous breasts as it is in modern cities, and every bit as dangerous.[20]

Moreover, the results of overcrowding are the same for breasts as they are for cities. In Victorian sociology, the slum is a mass of masses—Edwin Chadwick and others continually lump together its dirt ("masses of filth and offal" [166]) and its dirty bodies ("dense masses, scarcely covered" [163]) to make a single "pestilential mass" (80). In Victorian medical literature, cancerous masses metaphorically trash the breast, reducing it to a squalid area drowning in its own dirt.[21] Simply put, cancer grows out of a failure of cellular sanitation. Under normal conditions, the breast not only collects its garbage but also recycles it (the "waste products" of cells are subjected to "safe disposal or utilisation" [Creighton, *Contributions* 25]). But in cancer the heaped-up by-products of "reckless growth" (Paget, *Surgical Pathology* 696) contaminate the system, clogging its ducts (which "become extremely obstructed and dilated" [Sheild 316]), "overflowing" into surrounding areas (Creighton, *Contributions* 190), and flooding the breast itself with "the various cellular and fluid products of the imperfect secretion" (Creighton, *Contributions* 122).[22] In the slum, bad drainage results in a deadly buildup of matter: "Refuse, *debris*, and filth of every sort lies accumulating, festers and rots" (quoted in Engels 53), ultimately forming "a most foul and putrid mass, disgusting to the sight, and offensive to the smell" (quoted in Chadwick 91). Likewise, the breast's constitutional inability to flush out impurities transforms it into a sort of somatic sewer, a stinking stream of infectious filth: "pouring out an offensive ichor . . . composed of the *debris* of necrosed tissue," cancer rots out the foundations of the breast, leaving behind a "frightful . . . eroding" landscape of structural ruin and decay (Birkett 227). "Rotten, shreddy, and infiltrated" (Paget, *Surgical Pathology* 703), covered in "ragged, ir-regular ulcerations" (Nunn 118) and stinking with "dirty, foetid, brown-ish . . . discharge" (Nunn 54), the diseased breast is a disaster area, an inner city so degraded that it is even infested with rats, eaten away by "rodent ulcers."[23] Breast cancer might thus be said to generate a sort of "mass culture," an inherently unstable, inveterately social somatic state. As Le Bon himself puts it, "when the structure of a civilization is rotten, it is always the masses that bring about its downfall" (xviii).[24]

Given the palimpsestic quality of writing about urban squalor and diseased breasts, it should come as no surprise that the final figure in breast cancer's metonymic trajectory of decay is that of the prostitute. After all, the prostitute is the ultimate image of urban degradation, the woman who, in making her privates public, physically merges with the marketplace she is symbolically set against. Alexandre Parent-Duchâtelet writes that "prostitutes are just as inevitable in an urban district as are sewers, dumps, and refuse heaps. The authorities should take the same approach to each" (quoted in Reid 23). On a level with other trash, prostitutes are "mere masses of rottenness" (quoted in Walkowitz 151). Malignant masses are composed of similarly corrupt material, spreading themselves "promiscuously, in all the surrounding tissues within a certain area" (Paget, *Surgical Pathology* 699). Com-posed of "wandering elements" (Gross 16) that communicate their "infection" to "neighboring and distant parts" (Gross 28), cancer em-bodies on a cellular level what social critics described as "circulating harlotry" (Hemyng 476), the "daily occupation of spreading abroad . . . a contagious and deadly disorder" (Acton 73, ix).[25] Moreover, each situation is equally hopeless of cure: just as there is no way of perma-nently "extirpating the calling of the harlot" (Acton 9), so the "extirpa-tion" of the breast almost never prevents the recurrence of cancer: each is a "social plague that cannot be got rid of" (Acton 9), "a Pariah class existing within the bosom of society" (Acton 4).[26] Turning the social pathology of prostitution inside out, medicine described cancer as a form of fallenness arising from an industrial ruin within. Realizing a devastating conjunction between gender norms and urban forms, the cancerous breast is finally a kind of oversexed cesspool; a gaping hole with "pouting . . . lips" (Bryant 196) that not only "oozes" excess filth but also "weeps" (Birkett 216).

Descriptions of breast cancer thus map body and city onto one another, lumping them together in the image of the mass, a figure whose sheer materiality licenses a series of slippages between the slum and somatic space.[27] More specifically, the language of faulty "mass production" that surrounds breast cancer has the distinct effect of suggesting that cancer is not simply caused by modern economic patterns, but that in some essential, elemental way it contains them; that it replicates the degenerative trajectory of poorly managed economies in its very symptoms. Describing breast cancer as a version of the cultural process that was said to bring the disease about in the first place, medicine figures breast cancer as an industrial accident. Employing the imagery of political economy in the service of physiology, Victorian writing about breast cancer frames the breast's physical collapse as a conceptual one: the spread of unhealthy material takes shape as a corrupt, corrupting fall into material culture. As cancerous material takes on a life of its own, mechanically leveling distinctions between tissues ("primary tumours of the breast [are] nothing else than diseased breasts" [Creighton, *Contributions* 200]) and organs (in metastasis breast cells spread to the liver, the lungs, the brain, and the bones), the language used to describe this process of leveling amasses meaning by eroding constitutive distinctions between discrete physical forms. Tumors are the agents of this erosion, destroying both female flesh and the essential idea of that flesh—the notion that it possesses a substantive identity apart from the specific social forms of industrial modernity. Indeed, like the mob after which masses are modeled, the tumor's identity lies in its capacity to generate difference: the crowd "forms a single being . . . a new body possessing properties quite different from those of the bodies that have served to form it" (Le Bon 2, 6), while the mass has a "distinct individuality . . . there are the same differences among individual tumors as there are among individual persons" (Creighton, *Contributions* 180–81). In Victorian sociology, the notion of the mass effectively identified the poor with their surroundings; it referred equally to the city ("a mass of buildings" [Engels 361]), the pauper ("a mass of rags and filth" [Mayhew III:388]), the prostitute ("a mass of syphilis" [Acton 10]), and garbage ("a most foul and putrid mass" [quoted in Chadwick 91]), and so established a metonymic equivalency among them all. So, too, with cancer: cells and tissues are no longer themselves when they are brought together in the mass, and tumors consequently make bodily material over in the image of mass culture. Collapsing categorical distinctions between female bodies and factories, private and public spaces, medical models of breast cancer paradoxically render a physiological problem as an ontological one: cancer's wayward blending of body and city thus resolves into a kind of metonymic malignancy (the diseased breast is a city is a sewer is a slut), a massive series of elisions in which female flesh is (indecently) exposed as a cheap quantity wide open to any number of loose constructions (the mass is crowded with meanings; it is everything rolled into one).

It is tempting to see the linguistic patterning of breast cancer as a coded commentary on Victorian gender formation. Indeed, such an argument seems inevitable: we know that during the nineteenth century, the consolidation of a modern capitalist economy depended on binary oppositions between private and public spheres, oppositions that were made to seem natural in large part by the construction of the female body as essentially domestic, as biologically destined for motherhood.[28] And we can see how, in the discourse of breast cancer, these oppositions appear to break down. Where healthy breasts stand as synecdoches for femininity, diseased breasts take shape as deviations from sociosexual norms. Doing everything that women should not—going mad, going to work, going bad—cancerous breasts lose their distinctness *as* breasts, becoming instead anatomical analogues of precisely those social forms that were seen to be most hostile to proper femininity: crowds, slums, and prostitutes. It seems a logical, even necessary, step to conclude that there is an essential relation between the linguistic dimensions of breast cancer and broader social patterns, to suggest that in framing a specifically female disease in terms that were antithetical to cultural conceptions of femininity, medicine used the pathologically signifying breast to articulate more general anxieties about the status of female sexuality under capitalism.

Such an argument would run something like this: we would say that in using the material body as a metaphor for material culture—or rather, in using material culture as a metaphor for the material exigency of organic disease—the discourse of breast cancer described the female body as acutely unstable, incapable of maintaining either its health or its hermeneutic in the wake of economic development. And we would

read the discursive construction of cancer as a sickening gloss on prevailing social concerns about whether, and on what terms, a "pure"
femininity, apart from and uncorrupted by culture, could exist in an
emergent capitalist economy. Noting that the breast stands, finally, as a
point of imminent epistemological as well as anatomical collapse, a
material space whose ideological weight is utterly vulnerable to disease,
we would conclude that medicine used the multivalent notion of the
"mass" to simultaneously investigate the place of gender in an era of
growth, and to interrogate the concept of gender itself.

CRITICAL MASS

Or not. It's a sexy argument, the kind of thing that is often set forth
these days. But it is an argument that hinges on a series of extremely
problematic assumptions that I would like to take a few pages to lay out.
First, let me note that such an argument would necessarily depend on a
notion of breast cancer as a phenomenon that is ultimately meaningful
only insofar as it is about other things (specifically, about gender, mass
culture, and the vexed relation between the two). Let me note also that
in turning breast cancer into an allegory of Victorian culture, we wind
up learning what we already know: that scientific writing frequently
encodes distinct social and political agendas, that those agendas frequently revolve around a strategically unstable model of gender, and
that the Victorians were accomplished practitioners of such mystified
logic. And finally, let me note that such an interpretive move is the
trademark gesture of much Victorian writing about breasts themselves,
which locates the principal features of "woman" in the breast in order
to naturalize foregone conclusions about women's place in culture. It
makes me wonder: What, crucially, is the difference between a Victorian ideologue taking the breast as a synecdochal sign of femininity
and a postmodern feminist critic taking breast disease as the synecdochal sign of a wider cultural pathology, a pathology that has everything to do with the way Victorian femininity was framed? In ontological terms, I would suggest, not a lot. To argue that the cancerous breast
signaled the instability of gender in an emerging industrial economy
would be to accept some version of the very analogical patterns that I
am trying to critique.[29] The anachronistic quality of this logic becomes

all the more palpable when we recall that the target of such an analytical gesture is the Victorian reification of a restricted, restricting notion of woman.

The logical fallacy I am outlining here is far from hypothetical; indeed, it is a pattern that haunts a great deal of recent feminist thought, whose most basic intervention—that the idea of woman makes culture "work"—echoes the Victorian tendency to see its ideal woman as the heart and soul of culture. The Victorian woman and the woman posited by feminist theory are near relations—the one the cornerstone of an entire culture (the angel in the house), the other the cornerstone of an entire theory of culture (the angle in the house). So closely tied are they that it is often the Victorian woman who anchors work on gender and culture. Consider how many of the primary works of feminist scholarship are also primary works of Victorian studies—Kate Millett's *Sexual Politics* (1970) and Ellen Moers's *Literary Women* (1976) are two of the first works of feminist literary criticism; Martha Vicinus's anthologies *Suffer and Be Still* (1972) and *A Widening Sphere: Changing Roles of Victorian Women* (1977) helped inaugurate feminist historiography; and the feminist critique of science owes a foundational debt to Barbara Ehrenreich and Deirdre English's 1973 booklet, *Complaints and Disorders: The Sexual Politics of Sickness.*[30] Consider, too, how, in the wake of Foucault's largely theoretical "history" of Victorian sexuality, Anglo-American feminism's historical interest in Victorian culture began to include an interest in Victorian culture as a potential proving ground for contemporary gender theory.[31] When Joan Wallach Scott makes the nineteenth century into the occasion for theorizing "gender and the politics of history," or when Eve Kosofsky Sedgwick airs out Victorian closets with an eye toward developing an "axiomatic" of interpretive activism, the nineteenth century becomes a voyage into feminist methodology, a place to stage and work out certain problems in twentieth-century thinking about gender and sexuality.[32] Feminist critics have found in Victorian culture a chance to produce a literature of their own.

Much of this literature centers on the female body, whose sickly history shapes a political vision that takes Victorian ideology as an animating cause. In *Body/Politics: Women and the Discourses of Science* (1990), for example, editors Mary Jacobus, Evelyn Fox Keller, and Sally Shuttleworth explicitly cast feminist theory as a twentieth-century antidote to nineteenth-century gender ideology: "If nineteenth-century discourses cast the feminine body as the malfunctioning organism that embodies society's ills, twentieth-century discourses make the feminine body the site of its contradictory desires and social theories, including those of feminism itself" (9). The Victorian use of the female body as a microcosm for social dysfunction thus set the terms for all feminist work today: "In contemporary feminist theory, no issue is more vexed than that of determining the relations between the feminine body as a figure in discourse and as a material presence or biological entity" (3). A homology wrapped in an agenda, the mission articulated here inherits the form of the content it aims to critique. One result: the type of synecdochal reasoning that enabled Victorians to shape such figures as the prostitute or the hysteric as embodiments of social ills reappears in feminist critiques of late-twentieth-century body politics as a strategy for critiquing the reasoning of a culture that continues to place more pressure on the female body than it can fairly bear. The hysteric, reincarnated as a figure for female transgression, and the anorexic, whose symptoms have seemed variously to indict patriarchy, bourgeois ideology, mass culture, and even liberal humanism, are our most succinct expressions of this inheritance.[33] Just as Victorian models of gender naturalized women's roles by working from part to whole (a woman is her breasts, breasts are private, therefore women belong in private space), so recent work on "body politics" naturalizes arguments about the social construction of gender by making female symptoms into exemplary signs of "cultural politics."

   Nowhere is this logic more problematic than in feminist work on Victorian culture itself, where it can overdetermine arguments so thoroughly that at points they seem to collapse into their subject matter. Compare the Victorian model for how female bodies work with Mary Poovey's model for how texts work. Where the one is principally concerned with biological reproduction (its cultural work according to nineteenth-century gender ideology), the other is principally given over—just as inevitably—to "the reproduction of ideology" (its cultural work according to twentieth-century discourse theory): "Texts give the values and structures of values that constitute ideology body—that is, they embody them for and in the subjects who read" (*Uneven Developments* 17). Casting the text as the female body of cultural theory, Poovey generates a paradigm of signification that depends—like the culture she theorizes—on the essential fertility of the idea that female bodies carry and (pro)create meaning. Poovey's historical interest in Victorian debates about childbirth—the subject of chapter 2 of *Uneven Developments*—thus assumes a methodological significance, providing as it does the operative terms of her governing analogy: just as medical debates about reproduction "exposed the contradiction written into the Victorian image of woman" (25, 50), so "the conditions that govern the production of texts are reproduced in the texts themselves as the condition of possibility for meaning" (17). In *Other Women*, Anita Levy makes a similar move when she figures her scholarly project as a form of antiquarian psychotherapy. Situating herself as a sociological shrink whose job it is to uncover "material [that] is culturally rather than psychologically repressed" (4), she describes the labor of history writing as a form of hysterical transference between the analyst and her subject: "In the course of writing this book . . . I found that I was haunted in the still of the night at my desk by what I came to call, for want of a better word, demons. . . . I was haunted by all the things I hadn't said in this book, and by all the traces of the women whose thoughts and desires were suppressed in nineteenth-century England with the rise to power of the new middle classes" (3). For Levy, studying Victorian women involves becoming an academic version of one. Recognizing as part of her methodology the formal complicity that has historically mediated feminist scholarship, Levy imagines that responsible feminist research necessarily involves a problematic overidentification with the madwoman in the archive. As the vocabulary of nineteenth-century thinking about women's roles penetrates the analytical language of her twentieth-century critical counterpart, content naturalizes the form of its own analysis and the paradigms under examination begin to structure their own interpretation.

This tendency within feminist Victorian studies to reproduce analytical paradigms in the name of critiquing them may have something to do with a reliance on Victorian culture as both an archive and an origin, a means of doing history as a means of doing theory. In the cases of Poovey and Levy, this tension eventually resolves itself in a displacement of subject matter onto analytical form. Levy is more interested in a "woman with a discursive body" than in the bodies of actual women

(5); it is this discursive body that fuels Poovey's model, whose rigor relies on the figure of the text as a receptive ideological vessel. For both critics, then, producing a feminist account of what Poovey calls the "structural" psychology of Victorian culture involves replicating that psychology at the level of methodology (Poovey, *Uneven Developments* 19). I lay all this out because it is only after we see how some of the very logic that helped to produce essentialist ideas about sex is built into the concepts that contemporary feminist critics use to critique that logic that we can see how the argument about breast cancer sketched out in the previous section relies heavily on the unexamined anachronism of its own analytical terms.[34] It is based less on historical evidence than on historically determined elisions, and for that reason it is at once formulaic and flawed—predictable in the way it plugs its patterns into prefabricated models, and problematic in its failure to appreciate how closely tied those models are to the history they propose to illuminate. This is not to say that there is no argument to be made here, that breast cancer cannot be situated in a wider discursive and political context; nor even that breast cancer is not about gender in important, even decisive, ways. But it is to remark on the overwrought character of an argument whose founding premises may be said to be predicted—even scripted— by Victorian gender ideology. And it is to suggest that a species of categorical determinism that has its roots in Victorian gender ideology is built into the very foundations of academic feminism—so much so that even constructivist accounts of gender mirror some of the basic structural moves of Victorian essentialism. As content scripts form, form comes in turn to determine content, so much so that the sturdiest claim of Victorian culture—that woman, for better or worse, was essentially *womanly*, incapable of escaping her nature—finds a latter-day analogue in the most basic premise of feminist theory—that any discourse on the female body is essentially gendered, really incapable of signifying on other terms.[35]

My point is neither to malign gender as a category of analysis nor to impugn the project of feminist cultural theory—as a feminist analysis of Victorian medical literature, this chapter is deeply invested in each. Indeed, my aim is precisely to trace the limits of that investment: to make an argument about the history of breast cancer and to use breast cancer's recalcitrance (for it is as difficult to treat analytically as it is to treat clinically) to ask what we mean by feminist history in the first place. Working from the premise that any "history" comes into being only in writing—as a textual event, a product of reading—this chapter is ultimately an attempt to investigate the extent to which we create what we set out to find, an effort to probe the possibilities of a particular historical problem in order to lend insight into some of the more habitual gestures of contemporary thinking about gender and culture. More specifically, it is an exercise in close reading, an exploration of what happens to that all-too-stable concept of "history" when we take it seriously as a compilation of texts—texts whose special power it is to produce the firm effect of facts, of a world and time of real events that exist, simply and undeniably, outside of language.[36] These aims—to read breast cancer historically and to think history through breast cancer—are, I should add, deeply antagonistic to one another: it is difficult to make a historical argument when one is also busy arguing with the way historical arguments are frequently made. Even so, I pursue this course here because this analysis demands it. It is only through an anachronistic historicism that we may see how deeply committed to anachronism the Victorian discourse of breast cancer is in its own right.

The remainder of this chapter is thus devoted to rethinking the "evidence" assembled in the first section. As I noted above, the earlier argument depends on a dense confusion of material and method; it is a critique of analogy that proceeds analogically, an analysis of the cultural construction of an emblematic female body that takes that body to be an emblem of culture. As such, it reinscribes the conceptual patterns it discusses in the name of demystifying them. In what follows, I return to the language of breast cancer, reassessing both the inflection of that language and the context in which it was produced in order to offer an alternative reading of breast cancer's metaphoric "urbanity." Methodologically, I insist that before breast cancer is turned into a political allegory, it is crucial to let breast cancer be about itself—to listen more carefully to its language and to think more creatively about the work it does. When we attend more closely to the character of this language, particularly to its habit of making metaphor the basis of a resolutely rational prose, our picture of breast cancer's historical significance changes. Similarities between breast cancer and the language of political economy begin to

look like they may have more to do with genre—with the special difficulties inherent in generating and reading "objective" language—than
with gender construction per se.[37] Indeed, those similarities turn out
not to be analogies, but rather the space within which medicine developed a thoroughgoing critique of analogical thinking.

SECOND OPINION

Nineteenth-century medicine grounded much of its expertise in its
capacity to speak denotatively, to work within a language whose freedom from metaphor signified both its scientific seriousness and its
capacity for truth. This is spelled out most clearly by Rudolf Virchow,
the German physician and theorist who is remembered as the father of
cell theory.[38] Arguing that analogical thinking did more to impede
science than to advance it, Virchow devoted his career not simply to
studying physiology, but to studying how physiology was studied. He
was obsessed with how language inevitably shaped the thing it described, and worried in his lectures and writing about the difficulties
language thus posed for the development of a truly rational and responsible medical science. More specifically, Virchow worried about the
place of metaphor in scientific writing. According to Virchow, medicine is too willing to reason deductively, extrapolating facts from established theories rather than developing theories inductively, from close
observation of real material. In particular, he criticized the tendency of
much early nineteenth-century medical theory to reason analogically,
to draw conclusions about bodily processes by logically extending the
concepts that were used to describe those processes.[39] Such techniques
obfuscated the truth, shaping scientific perspective so thoroughly that
they actually impaired vision. The cell, for instance, was a new concept
not because scientists had only recently begun examining tissue under
the microscope (though improved lenses did revolutionize microscopy
during the 1820s), but because they literally could not see the structures
they were looking at. Without a notion of the cell, the cell was for all
practical purposes invisible. All too often, Virchow complained, theory
determined the facts rather than the other way around.[40] In response to
this lamentably inverted state of affairs, Virchow proposed a decep-
tively simple solution: a system of reasoning that sees knowledge as

originating in seeing itself. An outspoken proponent of positivism, Virchow sought to purify research by making close visual study the basis of all scientific theorizing. By replacing the syllogistic extravagance of contemporary medicine (if *x* then *y* then *z*) with a new, empirically derived standard of evidence, Virchow argued, medical science would be better able to approach the deep secrets he believed could be explained entirely in terms of that lone physical entity, the cell: "No matter how we twist and turn we shall always come back to the cell" (quoted in Rather, "The Place of Virchow's 'Cellular Pathology' in Medical Thought" xvi). "Beyond [cells] there is nothing but change" (Virchow, "Cellular Pathology" 85).

Simple enough in theory. But in practice, the means of replacing sloppy analogical thinking with a more rigorous logic of observation was less clear-cut. Indeed, even as Virchow presented empiricism as an antidote to a metaphorics of conjecture he was nonetheless entirely dependent on analogy as a technique of objective description. He often compared the organism to a little state, for example, describing it as a nation complete with class structure, healthy competition, and the occasional bad element whose well-being comes at the expense of the whole: "What is an organism? A society of living cells, a tiny well-ordered state, with all the accessories—high officials and underlings, servants and masters, the great and the small. . . . As in the lives of nations, so in the lives of individuals the state of health of the whole is determined by the well-being and close interrelation of the individual parts; disease appears when individual members begin to sink into a state of inactivity disadvantageous to the commonwealth, or to lead parasitic existences at the expense of the whole" ("Atoms and Individuals" 130, 139). How are we to understand this paradox? First, we have to recognize that Virchow is careful to keep analogy secondary to observation, using it to illustrate what he has observed to be true rather than as a technique of inference. He has not deduced the existence of cells from what he knows of states, but has seen cells under the microscope and seeks to describe them by comparison with a known quantity. Second, and more important, we must consider how Virchow's inversion of cause and effect—using analogy as a mechanism for reporting what he has seen rather than as a strategy for generating things to see—involves a fundamental revision of analogy itself. In Virchow's hands, analogies work, paradoxically, to assert difference, drawing parallels between separate things in order to drive home the incomparable particularity of living systems. His interest in the individual/state analogy, for instance, is precisely its failure to capture a likeness: "Nothing resembles life except life itself," he writes; "The state can be termed an organism, since it consists of living citizens; conversely the organism can be termed a state, or a family, since it consists of living members of like origin. But here the comparison is at an end" (130). Life is incomparable, unlike anything else. And for this reason it both cannot be described in terms of other things and must be, if it is to be described at all.

Virchow's ongoing flirtation with the state as a metaphor for living systems points neither to a myopic lack of self-awareness nor to a grandiose belief in his own exemption from the practice he preaches. Rather, it must be read as a highly ingenious way of negotiating the defining paradox of the genre in which he is writing: that as much as analogies threaten to obscure the truth of bodily systems, it is necessary to draw them if the truth about life is to be told. Virchow's preface to *Cellular Pathology* (1858) notes that the very success of empiricism has created a language barrier within medicine:

> Day by day do those who are obliged to consume their best energies in the frequently so toilsome and so exhausting routine of practice find it becoming less and less possible for them, not only to closely examine, but even to understand the recent medical works. For even the language of medicine is gradually assuming another appearance; well-known processes to which the prevailing system had assigned a certain place and name in the circle of our thoughts, change with the dissolution of the system their position and their denomination. When a certain action is transferred from the nerves, blood, or vessels to the tissues, when a passive process is recognized to be an active one, an exudation to be a proliferation, then it becomes absolutely necessary to choose other expressions whereby these actions, processes, and products shall be designated; and in proportion as our knowledge of the more delicate modes, in which the processes of life are carried on, becomes more perfect, just in that proportion must the new denominations also be adapted to this more delicate ground-work of our knowledge. (6)

It is not just that new observations require new language, Virchow notes, but that this language is itself in need of observation: unwatched, its very precision becomes a means of obfuscation, something whose increasing exactness makes it fundamentally unclear. Virchow's mission, in *Cellular Pathology* and elsewhere, is to ensure the accessibility of medicine to its practitioners, to discover a language of description that not only allows detailed accounts of bodily processes to make sense, but that also enables those accounts to keep up with the times, to be sensibly revised and particularized as new and better techniques for studying anatomy and physiology are developed. To that end, he embraces analogy anew. The proper way to describe new things (cells), Virchow's prose asserts, is to compare them to what is already known (states); in other words, the way to develop an accessible language based on observation is to borrow already familiar language from elsewhere. That language, moreover, should be obviously inexact, incapable of withstanding careful scrutiny. Like the individual/state comparison, good analogies should crumble under pressure, exposing otherwise incommunicable truths through the force of their own false comparisons.

For Virchow, then, a proper analogy does less to establish a genuine likeness between separate entities than it does to mark the sheer difficulty involved in establishing the singular identity of individual entities. In other words, analogy is Virchow's concession to the very real problems inherent in generating a useful scientific vocabulary, his acknowledgment that rational, objective discourse cannot fairly proceed in the absence of the very thing from which it seeks to differentiate itself: metaphor. Without analogy there is only tautology: "*Life is cell activity; its uniqueness is the uniqueness of the cell*" ("On the Mechanistic Interpretation of Life" 106; original emphasis). With analogy there exists, paradoxically, the possibility of naming. Cells can signify themselves as cells only after they have been compared—reductively—to states. Likewise, abnormal growths of cells become analytically accessible only when they are named after other things.

Virchow's example of such comparative anatomy is the "colloid tumor," a common kind of growth characterized by a soft, sticky interior. The name *colloid*, Virchow notes, "was invented at the commencement of the present century by Laennec to designate a form of tumour which he described as analogous in consistence to half-set glue; in its well-developed form it constitutes a half-trembling jelly, colourless or of slightly yellowish hue, which on the whole conveys the impression of a nearly complete absence of all structure" (*Cellular Pathology* 510). But Virchow rejects the term even so; such names are inaccessible, he objects, "nothing more than stop-gags":

> Whilst people formerly declared themselves perfectly content, when tumours of this kind were designated jelly-like, or gelatinous, to many of the more recent observers it has appeared a proof of superior penetration to say, instead of gelatinous tumour or gelatinous mass, colloid tumour or colloid mass. But you must not think that those, who have these denominations the most constantly in their mouths, intend to express anything else by them, than what most others call simply a jelly-like tumour, or only jelly. . . . It is, however, very advisable, that these really unmeaning and only high-sounding expressions should not be unnecessarily diffused, and that the habit should be acquired of conveying a precise meaning by every expression, and that therefore from the moment one really aspires to make histological divisions, one should no longer employ, when speaking of every jelly-like tumour, the term colloid which has no histological value whatever, but merely designates an external appearance which tissues of the most different nature may under certain circumstances present. (510–11)

Colloid is a useless term, annoyingly obscure and, as a consequence, scientifically inexact, a formal designation that lumps together growths of different origins: "The chief difficulty, which here presents itself, consists in this, that people do not know how to discover any difference between *the mere form and the true nature*" (511; original emphasis). A more proper name for colloid can be found, ironically, by reverting to medicine's time-honored tradition of analogical thinking, and calling it after something else: "a jelly-like tumour, or only jelly." The result is to prefer the rich association of a wrong name to the empty denotation of an expressly scientific term: since the stuff inside colloid tumors is *like* jelly, Virchow suggests, it is more precise to talk about them as tumors filled *with* jelly than it is to call them colloids.

Virchow's desire to reduce colloids to jellies demonstrates not simply a distrust of slick scientific vocabulary, but a belief that a better science lies in a strategically inexact language. *Colloid* means nothing—it is an ontological vacuum, incapable of connoting. But jelly *is* something, a misnomer so palpably impossible that it operates denotatively, serving as a perfectly precise name for the thing it describes. (A sweet irony: *colloid* is no less analogical than *jelly*. From the Greek *kollo*, meaning "glue," Laennec's proper name for this sort of growth is every bit as metaphorical as the analogy that replaced it. The difference is simply one of accessibility. Colloid's metaphorical dimensions are so obscure that in practical terms they do not exist.) Ironically, then, Virchow's pursuit of reference led him to embrace analogy as a viable mode of medical description. His antidote for medicine's tendency to reason analogically is to replace it with an elaborately associative poetics of observation, a poetics that crucially does not always announce itself as such. For example, in converting colloid tumors to jellylike tumors to simple jelly, Virchow moves from proper name to metaphor to catachresis, from a name-that-conceals-analogy to an analogy-that-acts-as-a-name. The effect is paradoxical, to say the least: jelly can be an identity because it is the most palpable analogy; it is the most referential way to discuss colloid tumors because it refers so successfully to what it is not.

Virchow's digressions on language provide a necessary framework for reading the specific analogical patterns associated with breast cancer. They make visible the sheer linguistic difficulty of developing a properly scientific discourse of the body, showing up the problems nonmetaphoric language posed for sense making at the same time that they show how densely metaphorical all language ultimately is. And they allow us to see how, in the context of a newly modern, increasingly positivist medicine, talking about disease—or any physiological process—was an inherently analogical project, a constant struggle to explain what was literally unheard of in language that was not only precise but palpably clear. Exactness demanded allusion; naming new things necessitated an initial naming-after. Read in this light, breast cancer's symbolic economy begins to look less like a simple case of covert analogy and more like a complex technique of description in which analogies are ranged, paradoxically, in direct opposition to analogical thinking.

Consider first how breast cancer's images take shape. At once totally

there and totally submerged, the language of production and degeneration that circulates through Victorian writing about breast cancer never
announces itself as such. Instead, it manifests itself as single words and
phrases scattered across texts, repeated often but at random, never set
off as a reference to or comparison with another sort of production;
indeed, never set off as figurative at all. In short, the economic affect of
medical writing about breast cancer appears, like Virchow's jelly, in the
guise of catachresis, as a mass of words that ought to be metaphors but
are instead the only words for the things they describe. Breast cancer
produces fruit clusters and crowded neighborhoods as accurate descriptors. Strung seamlessly into measured prose, they are allusive enough to
make meaning, but not apt (in the absence of a late twentieth-century
critical sensibility) to link breast cancer to anything but itself.

Breast cancer's professed objectivity thus depends on a very precise
imprecision: while the descriptive languages of Victorian mass culture
are everywhere present in the discourse of breast cancer, those languages are never actually identified as such. What is missing in the
language of breast cancer is the moment of making explicit; in other
words, the moment of intentionality, of ownership. The language of the
factory system becomes the language of breast cancer, but at no point is
the breast actually compared to a factory. Nor are the commodity, the
prostitute, or the slum ever named as such. Their vocabularies supply
the descriptive needs of breast cancer only insofar as their characteristic
words and phrases are detached from their original points of reference.
While terms associated with production and waste, surplus and decay,
poverty, promiscuity, and mass violence enable some of breast cancer's
most vivid descriptions, those terms depend for their success on a strategic dislocation. Explicit comparisons would ground that vocabulary
firmly in a logic of comparison by locating them as the rhetoric of urban
space. Underrealized analogies, by contrast, create the necessary conditions for a self-contained language of description by allowing medicine
to subsume an enormously provocative part—the breast—within an
orderly analytical whole. Cancerous breasts do not refer to the world
beyond them; they simply adapt its attendant descriptors, using them
to generate a new set of references having to do with tumor formation,
metastasis, and recurrence.

In order to see how this may be so, we must take a moment to consider the phenomenon of catachresis more closely than we have done so far. By definition, catachresis marks a fragment of nonmeaning; it is a figure that does not do the work of figuration. Even if it is part of a series, catachresis is always isolated and alone. This is true of medical writing about breast cancer, where the patterns I have described multiply within and across texts but do not grow. They appear over and over, but they never build, evolve, or connect. They do not know they are there, and they never add up to anything more than themselves— although they may sometimes seem to. As such, catachresis describes a most difficult and resistant sort of text. It is pure surface, reflection without depth. Its genuine aim is to describe, never to compare. And as such, it finally signifies limitation, eliminating movement in the moment of figuration, and so making of approximation a proper name for the thing. Less is more in catachresis; catachresis is language that is not all it seems to be.

As resonant as Victorian writing about breast cancer is, then, it cannot quite be called allusive: its metaphors go nowhere; they are substitutes for a set of ideal referents that do not exist. So, while the language of political economy is very much there in breast cancer, it is not there *as such*. Rather, it is there as breast cancer's own special vocabulary of objective description. Ranged in the service of mimesis, breast cancer's metaphors constitute the stuff of a nascent neutrality: they are simply "the" language of cancer itself. Consequently, any echoes we hear between the two spaces are incidental: not only are they not actually meant to mean, they are there in order *not* to mean.[41] The gesture of catachresis is one of emptying, of keeping the sign while definitively altering the signified. As form with new content, sign utterly severed from its original sense, catachresis culminates in a nonmetaphoric effect: it specifically satisfies the drive of medical description to achieve a pure referentiality. Far from encouraging a set of fraught associations across ideologically apposite spaces, it seems, breast cancer's cultural allusions are there in the name of proper naming. Aiming not to align its constituents but to capture the essence of one by appropriating the sense of the other, the discourse of breast cancer borrows the language of political economy not in order to compare breasts to cities, but rather in order not to be comparative at all. In a stunning reversal of cause and effect, breast cancer's metaphors paradoxically enable that overdetermined organ to operate—for once—as a point of perfect self-reference, to be simply and absolutely about itself.

This is not to say that gender is not an important factor in Victorian conceptualizations of breast cancer. As we have seen, the perceived causes of breast cancer were tied closely to the presumed difficulty women had in accommodating themselves to the particular stresses of modern civilized life. And we have seen how the belief that breast cancer came from a specifically modern emotional imbalance filtered through medical representations of cancer's early phases, leading physicians to describe breast cancer as the result of cellular hysteria, a microscopic inability to manage life with potentially fatal results. But it is to say that in the realm of medical theory there was a specific move to separate the breast from sex, by separating it from the kinds of connotations it held elsewhere. And it is to say that it was precisely through the vocabulary of sanitary reform that medicine effected this ontological maneuver. This language was in itself densely metaphorical and deeply political, committed to anatomizing social crisis by way of that provocative abstraction, the social body.[42] But in the context of medical description, the language of the city operates paradoxically as a way of decoupling breasts and sex, as a way of converting the fraught territory of female sexuality into a neutral analytical zone. Detaching the breast from an identifiably gendered vocabulary and grounding it in a language that has the double advantage of apparent descriptive neutrality (early sociology participated in the new empirics of observation) and complete incommensurability (sociology was centered on culture, not cancer), the language of breast cancer dematerializes the breast, abstracting it from the kinds of conceptual operations that organ was wont to fulfill—so much so that even seemingly damning analogies between breasts and such degraded social entities as prostitutes and crowds do not register as analogies, do not come off as loaded comparisons. As such, the cancerous breast becomes the basis for a sort of ideological neutering. In framing the cancerous breast as the city's catachresis, medicine managed to shape that organ as neither breast nor city. Instead, it rendered the breast profoundly nonassociative, a point of reference whose principal reference point is simply and only itself.

My point here is not only to note how closely tied cancer has been, since the nineteenth century, to both analogical thinking and a critique of analogical thinking, but also to register the methodological implications of such a realization. For once we recognize Victorian medicine's deeply ambivalent and immensely innovative relationship to analogy for what it is, both our understanding of Victorian medical history and our techniques for illuminating that history fall into doubt. We cannot, for example, simply assume that the metaphors submerged within the discourse of breast cancer tell a story of unexamined gender ideology masquerading as objective truth. As accepted as such an argument has come to be—it is, after all, one of the founding ideas in the feminist critique of science—it does not work here for the simple reason that we cannot read the cancerous breast as a sign of Victorian medicine's abiding culturalism without indulging in the same sorts of analogical extrapolations that medicine was itself increasingly coming to understand as evidence of faulty logic and bad scientific faith.[43] The linguistic patterns surrounding breast cancer thus pose a peculiar problem for feminist historiography: once we approach its metaphors as a technique of mimesis, we have also to recognize that breast cancer is not so much an unwitting discourse about gender as it is a discourse that is doing its level best not to be about gender at all. The question, then, is not, How does the discourse of breast cancer construct gender? but rather, How does the discourse of breast cancer *elide* gender? How does it produce a discursive situation in which the breast ceases to be the very sign of sex and becomes instead the scene of objective referentiality?

The answer should not surprise us, given what we have learned about the capacity of medical language to fill old forms with new content. Just as Virchow gave colloid meaning by converting it to jelly, so medicine emptied the breast of its sexual content by simply filling it up with a new set of symbolic associations. The discourse of breast cancer relies on synecdoche to elide femininity: the breast ceases to be an emblem of womanhood when it becomes a microcosm of metastatic disease. Clinically, breast cancer upset doctors. Until the introduction of the radical mastectomy in the 1890s, breast cancer was a disease doctors could do little to manage and nothing to cure. And that meant that they had routinely to watch women die ugly, painful deaths. Theoretically, though, the situation was somewhat different. What made breast cancer so interesting to doctors was not so much that it happened almost exclusively to women, but that it could illustrate so many of the laws governing metastatic disease. Breast cancer was both a common form of cancer and a cancer that took a range of forms. Scirrhous breast cancers were hard, poorly circumscribed, and painful; medullary cancers appeared as round lumps, movable but not wholly separate from surrounding tissue; fibroplastic, or colloid, cancers, as we have seen, were slow growing, deep, and became spongy and gelatinous over time. Breast cancers could be fast-growing, soft, and painless; or slow, hard growths with shooting pains. Some spread fast and killed quickly, others lay dormant for years while their victims led relatively normal lives. Some looked like cysts, others like sores; some were so small as to be virtually undetectable; others grew huge or simply ate away the breast. Breast cancer was, in short, great material—so varied, so chronically different from itself, that it came as close as any single form of cancer could to reproducing all the forms that cancer could take. Indeed, the very quality that made breast cancer difficult to grasp clinically—its sheer variability—made it a wonderful foil for theory: taken in its entirety, breast cancer amounted to a remarkably typical form of metastatic disease. To talk about breast cancer was thus always also to talk more generally about the phenomenon of cancer.

As such, breast cancer became a privileged site for theorizing cancer: in the depths of theory, breast cancer is seen not so much as a disease that is localized in women, but rather as a disease that localizes cancer itself. James Paget's elaborate analysis of cancer in *Surgical Pathology* is a case in point. For Paget, breast cancer exemplifies so many of the classic patterns of cancerous depletion that it cannot be confined to the section on "Mammary Glandular Tumors" (484–91). Interested more in cancer as a phenomenon than in the cancers of specific organs, he weaves references to breast cancer throughout his study of tumors and the different types of cancer. A few examples of breast cancer's exemplary behavior: under the category of "Fibrous Cancer," it is "one of the best marked cases in which a tumor, presenting the usual characters of a fibrous tumor, not only recurred after removal, but even formed secondary tumors of a like nature in internal organs" (665); under "Scirrhous or Hard Cancer," the breast is mentioned first "because here the disease is far more frequent than in any other part, and presents, openly, most of its varieties of appearance according to its successive stages, and the accidents to which it is exposed" (520). Elsewhere, the breast demonstrates the myeloid tumor's occasional malignancy (470) and the "accidental proximity" of malignant and benign growths: "a scirrhous cancer may occupy part of a mammary gland, in the rest of which are many cysts that are in no sense cancerous" (663). Where Paget finds that cancer is often best discussed in terms of breast cancer, Willard Parker's 1885 inquiry into the causes of cancer sees breast cancer as a representation of cancer generally. Relying on 397 cases of breast cancer as his primary source of data, Parker extrapolates the general laws of cancer entirely from the specific pathological patterns of cancerous breasts. Both men see breast cancer as a synecdochal pathology whose knotty particulars double as generalizations and whose specifics are grossly characteristic. At once unmistakably itself and absolutely emblematic, breast cancer is symptomatic of cancer as a whole. Conceptually, then, breast cancer continually slips away: its symptoms are always signs of something else; its material reality is always also a potential point of reference. Sliding imperceptibly into a broader philosophical inquiry into the nature of metastatic disease, breast cancer is ultimately a textbook pathology, a materialization of what would otherwise remain something of an abstraction.

Breasts colluded in their own abstraction. Doctors struggled to define what the breast was, where it began and ended. It was a gland without obvious boundaries, an organ that was essentially contiguous with surrounding tissues. (This sense of the breast as a fundamentally fuzzy or indefinite part is exemplified in our tendency to use the terms *breast* and *chest* interchangeably.) Cancer made the ill-defined nature of the breast painfully visible, spreading so readily to surrounding tissue and bone that surgical protocols increasingly argued that the breast could not be fully removed without also excising axillary glands and pectoral muscle. In so doing, breast cancer showed a breast that was not really there. Outlining an organ that could be localized only if it included organs outside itself (muscle, lymph nodes), breast cancer revealed the breast itself as an abstraction, an anatomical ideal that disappears the moment it is subjected to scrutiny. And breast cancer was itself a peculiarly textual pathology in which breast tissue ceases to signify itself, and instead begins to be representative of other things. In his *Contributions to the Physiology and Pathology of the Breast*, Charles Creighton describes the diseased breast as inherently mimetic: the na-

ture of breast cancer is to "copy" (186) and "mimic" (180) the look of
other things. Tumors "can hardly be admitted to be things in themselves" (178), Creighton asserts, but are, rather, vehicles for the transformation of one sort of material into another: "There is indeed an infinite
variety of appearances in the pathological mammary structure; there is
nothing of it, one may say, but is changed into 'something rich and
strange'" (127). For Creighton, cancer is a process by which the breast
accumulates a wealth of representations: the "strangeness" of the cancerous breast is synonymous with its "richness," but what the breast is
rich in is "appearances." Creighton suggests that the reality of the disease is that it never simply exists as such—in assuming an "infinite
variety of appearances," the cancerous breast always seems to be something other than what it actually is.

So it is that Victorian medical writing about breast cancer charts not
the progressive destruction of gender as such, but the gradual erasure of
gender as a determining factor in the significance of a woman's disease.
Infusing the breast with a rhetoric that is ideologically opposed to all
the breast stands for works not to denaturalize the breast (by polluting
its separate sphere) but to neutralize it, to stop the spread of association,
the automatic linking of breast to sex, and sex to social role. Formal
conflation was, ironically, a way of emptying both categories of specific
referential content: the linguistic collapse of the female body and the
inner city was very decidedly not a conceptual collapse. The special
triumph of this discourse is the neutral effect it achieves through the
elimination of connotation. Objectivity, in the discourse of breast cancer, emerges out of a language that is at once deeply connotative and
absolutely removed from its figural roots, legible only as pure denotation. Rather than working to implicate a woman's private disease in the
problems afflicting the public sphere, the discourse of breast cancer
decontextualizes the breast and so transforms the symbol of woman
into a neutral conceptual zone, a place not for thinking gender but for
thinking "cancer."

The immediate intellectual payoff is clear enough: medicine gains a
useful conceptual figure, a synecdoche for cancer and a way to protect
the fragile synecdoches of femininity from the signal erosions of cancer.
For those are what must be sheltered from cancer, what must not be in
play when real disease destroys the sign of a woman's femininity. Else

the sort of reasoning I proposed originally—the reading of breast cancer's urbanity as a kind of embodied destruction of femininity—would
be in operation; else breast cancer's process would *mean*, would indicate
a fatal flaw with gender itself. But such was hardly the aim of Victorian
medical writing; rather, the simultaneous reduction of the breast to a
cipher of the city and the conflation of the cancerous breast with cancer
must be read as a mode of abstraction, a means not of debunking breasts
by grounding them critically in their social contexts, but of creating
them as conceptually removed spaces, areas whose immediate significance comes directly from their apparent symbolic isolation.

Medicine's abstracted breasts were not mere symbolic niceties, a way
of erasing the awful reality of a woman's disease. They were, rather,
what enabled medicine to approach breast cancer as a problem to be
solved, and so to work steadily toward a cure. At midcentury, the prospect of curing breast cancer was so bleak that prominent surgeons such
as James Syme (the surgeon who operated on the real-life Ailie) and
James Paget were publicly voicing their opinion that it was useless even
to attempt to treat cancer. Too many women died under the knife or of
complications following surgery (de Moulin 79); and it was doubtful
that those who survived lived even as long as women who went un-
treated (Paget's research showed that women operated on for scirrhous
cancer of the breast died an average of thirteen months earlier than
women who did not undergo surgery [de Moulin 80]). Surgery for
breast cancer was fast becoming an empty form: the well-known Philadelphia surgeon Hayes Agnew even admitted that although he had no
hope that surgery would lengthen the life of a woman with breast
cancer, he sometimes operated anyway for the patient's morale. This
hopeless mood was complicated by a widespread inability to separate
the diseased breast from the woman to whom it was attached. As Samuel Warren put it in 1830, breast cancer illustrated "the great firmness of
the female sex, and [its] powers of enduring a degree of physical pain
which would utterly break down the stubborn strength of man" (474).
Warren's article in *Blackwood's* tells the story of a woman's mastectomy
as the story of her feminine forbearance. A "victim of that terrible
scourge of the female sex—a cancer," Mrs. St——'s cancer is deeply
rooted in her sexuality; "an eminent medical writer has remarked that
the most beautiful women are generally the subjects of this terrible

disease," Warren remarks (474–75). Written from the perspective of "a late physician," the column recounts how the narrator's insistent gendering of Mrs. St——'s cancer, his inability to distance the diseased breast from a sense of her sex, caused him no end of professional difficulty. Overcome by the sight of the "hateful instruments" and his own "agitated air," he winds up moaning and quaking much like a woman himself: "Was it this innocent and beautiful being who was doomed to writhe beneath the torture and disfigurement of the operating knife? My heart ached. . . . I could scarce avoid a certain nervous tremor—unprofessional as it may seem" (474–75). Until the latter half of the nineteenth century, breast cancer was not only largely fatal but also overwhelmingly feminine: the combination was unnerving for physicians, who were both professionally and personally helpless before it.[44]

The introduction of cellular pathology, anesthesia, and antisepsis definitively changed the face of breast cancer. During the last quarter of the century, survival rates for mastectomy went steadily up: Billroth reported that between 1867 and 1875, 4.7 percent of his cases lived for three years or more; in 1877, Banks reported a 20 percent survival rate; and in 1894, Halsted reported that 45 percent of his breast cancer patients lived for at least three years after mastectomy.[45] The reasons for these increasing rates were twofold. First, improved technology allowed surgeons to improve their craft (whereas speed and minimal disruption of tissue were of essence in the era before anesthesia, the scrupulous mastectomies performed by Halsted at the turn of the century would sometimes last for four to five hours). Second, surgeons were removing progressively more and more flesh in their effort to remove all traces of cancer from the affected area (as one surgeon put it: "If the disease recurs so frequently why not cut deeper?" [Sweeting 323]). Billroth achieved his 4.7 percent survival rate by performing simple mastectomies: all he removed was the breast tissue itself. Banks and others quadrupled Billroth's rates by routinely removing axillary glands as well as the diseased breast. And Halsted justified the most invasive procedure yet—the complete removal of breast, underlying pectoral muscle, and axillary glands known as the radical mastectomy—with his unprecedented rates of cure.[46] And so it was that breast cancer went from a hopeless cause—a "dreadful and poignant malady" (Butter 507), "that terrible scourge of the female sex" (Warren 474)—to a manageable condition in the space of twenty-five years, a historic development that was oweing in no small part to the rhetorical separation of breast and sex evident in medical writing from midcentury on.

Neutralizing the breast in writing made it possible to contemplate breast cancer as a surgical rather than a sexual problem; made it possible to experiment with operative techniques, to debate the relative merits of partial and total extirpations, to develop techniques for removing surrounding tissues, to find the most efficient type of cut, and to shape the healthiest wound. The result: physicians relinquished aesthetic concerns (a desire to preserve as much of the breast as possible, especially the nipple, had dominated breast cancer treatment since the late eighteenth century) and learned to see the cancerous breast as something far removed from questions of sexuality, identity, and womanhood. As Samuel Gross put it in 1880, "The management of mammary neoplasms should be based solely upon the conclusions drawn from the prominent facts in their life, which we have now learned in studying their general pathology" (82). In 1830, Samuel Warren's inability to detach his professional interest in Mrs. St——'s breast cancer from his true awe of her beauty and goodness made it hard for him to treat her. In 1880, Samuel Gross displayed a detachment so complete that the only life affecting his medical decisions was the life of the cancer itself. Objectifying, yes: but only as a saving grace.[47]

PROGNOSIS FOR A FEMINIST CRITIQUE OF SCIENCE

Much recent feminist work on scientific language has centered on how its presumed "neutrality" is never neutral and has devoted its energies to elaborating how ostensibly objective language almost always encodes political claims about gender, class, and race. Generally speaking, such critiques read metaphor *as* metaphor, as definite if unself-conscious moments of descriptive lapse that are dangerously susceptible to becoming "naturalized" and so "disguised" (Stepan 125). As a generic Freudian slip, metaphor functions in most of this work as a window to ideology: it is in gendered metaphors that we can read the political underpinnings of supposedly objective work. The focus is on "the inhibitory costs of gendered metaphors," on the capacity of metaphor to impair scientific progress by "lending certain kinds of processes an aura of unthinkability" (Keller and Longino 6–7). Locating metaphors as moments of nonscience, this body of work reads figural language as the point at which we can see culture intruding most invidiously into scientific thought—it is there that we can begin to unfurl the deeply subjective assumptions that figure into and help frame "objectivity." The assumption is that metaphors are moments of mystification: they either don't know they are there (most metaphors show up in scientific descriptions by accident) or don't know they are metaphors (some metaphors pass themselves off as statements of fact).[48] Either way, metaphors figure as signs of science's lack of neutrality, and they direct us to the particular nature of its hidden biases.

This chapter has undertaken a more elemental project. Rather than expose the gendered meanings underlying scientific formulations, it seeks to understand how "gender" itself came to be hidden (came to be a category to be hidden) in the first place, how gender came somehow not to figure as the determining analytical category for doctors attempting to understand what breast cancer was and how it could be cured. Instead of simply reading breast cancer's urban metaphors as signs of medicine's failure to be neutral, this chapter reads those metaphors as the place where medicine actively constructed itself as neutral, treating the cancerous breast as a conceptually overdetermined ground on which the phenomenon of neutrality was being actively invented and explored. Such an approach forces us to reexamine both the content of Victorian medical discourse and our present strategies for writing about it. We tend to treat Victorian scientists—particularly doctors—as largely naive about the ideological dimensions of their own pretensions to objectivity, and have understood our job, consequently, as one of correction, of pointing out how densely political medical language inevitably was and still is—particularly in its handling of marginal groups such as women, criminals, people of color, the insane, and the poor. But once we see how troubled medicine could be by the difficulties involved in finding a descriptive language that was not loaded with cultural associations, we have to reconsider not only what the language of the city is doing in descriptions of breast cancer, but what we are doing when we set out to analyze it. More specifically, studying breast cancer forces us to consider catachresis as a historical, textual, and analytical entity. For the phenomenon of the metaphor-as-referent, the allusion that does not allude, cannot properly register within an analytical climate that thinks culture almost exclusively by forging meaningful connections across disparate discursive spaces and treats figurative language as a guide to a given text's "political unconscious." Thinking catachresis in turn forces us to think more carefully about what constitutes "context," and about what we mean when we say that signifying practices are "political."

There is a vast body of work dedicated to showing how, since the nineteenth century, the female body has enabled certain social conformations to seem natural; how biology has been used to mystify "gender" as "sex," and so to essentialize cultural concepts of woman. This chapter takes up a particular strand of that history, a strand that does not fit—though, crucially, it initially appears to—in order to point up some of the dangers inherent in this analytical project. For if Victorians did map gender onto sex, finding justification for women's roles in their brains, breasts, wombs, and cells, they also sought at points not to do this, to remove the female body from precisely the kinds of overdetermined associations that it was otherwise so instrumental in framing. Likewise, just as feminist and cultural critics have set themselves the task of uncovering the ideological dimensions of textual patterns, combating essentialist formations by exposing them as interested cultural constructions, so too do they run the risk of essentializing ideology itself, of assuming the "political nature" of certain textual patterns without fully assessing the terms on which those patterns are formed and the contexts in which they are framed. In this respect, we might say that if the patterns I chart in the language of breast cancer mark anything, they mark the extreme limit—or limitation—of our own techniques for thinking culture. They make visible the reductive potential inherent in the otherwise important realization that culture works through texts in ways authors did not necessarily control or even know about. And they raise pressing questions about what we mean when we say—as we do with increasing ease—that the body is a cultural signifier. Ultimately, then, the case of breast cancer urges us to investigate the extent to which we create what we set out to find. In its inability to sustain the sort of reading we are increasingly representing as historical knowledge, it raises far more basic questions about where knowledge comes from and what new ways of knowing might be available to us, if only we would learn to look for them.

THREE

Fractions of Men: Engendering Amputation

In 1866, the *Atlantic Monthly* published a fictional case study of an army surgeon who had lost all of his limbs during the Civil War. Written anonymously by the American neurologist Silas Weir Mitchell, "The Case of George Dedlow" describes not only the series of wounds and infections that led to the amputation of all four of the soldier's arms and legs, but also the aftereffects of amputation. Reduced to what he terms "a useless torso, more like some strange larval creature than anything of human shape," Dedlow finds that in disarticulating his body, amputation articulates anatomical norms. His observation of his own uniquely altered state qualifies him to speak in universal terms about the relationship between sentience and selfhood: "I have dictated these pages," he says, "not to shock my readers, but to possess them with facts in regard to the relation of the mind to the body" (5). As such, the story explores the meaning of embodiment, finding in a fragmented anatomy the opportunity to piece together a more complete understanding of how the body functions—physically and metaphysically—as a whole.[1]

In Mitchell's story, amputation disrupts the relationship between body and mind, and consequently undermines Dedlow's sense of self. Noting that after the loss of his limbs he needs very little food and hardly any sleep, and that even his resting heart rate has slowed from seventy-eight to forty-five beats per minute, Dedlow associates the depression of his vital functions with a parallel mental decline. He suffers most from what he calls "a deficiency in the egoistic sentiment of individuality," a "want of being myself." Blaming his emotional deficiencies on his anatomical ones, he explicitly links the absence of his limbs to an increasing absence of mind: "About one half of the sensitive surface of my skin was gone, and thus much of [my] relation to the outer world destroyed. As a consequence, a large part of the receptive central organs must be out of employ, and, like other idle things, degenerating rapidly. Moreover, all the great central ganglia, which give rise to movements in the limbs, were also eternally at rest. Thus one half of me was absent or functionally dead. This set me to thinking how much a man might lose and yet live" (8).

For Dedlow, amputation provides a depressingly precise confirmation of mid-Victorian physiological tenets. Henry Maudsley writes in *Body and Mind* (1871) that we "must recognize how entirely the integrity of the mental functions depends on the integrity of the bodily organization." In Dedlow's case, this dependence can be calibrated: the integrity of his mind is directly proportional to the integrity of his body (94–95).[2] Positing an almost arithmetical dependence of subjectivity on the senses, he argues that when the body is incomplete, personality is partial too: "A man is not his brain, or any one part of it, but all of his economy, and . . . to lose any part must lessen this sense of his own existence" (8). In Mitchell's story, the pathology of amputation can be absolutely quantified—the degree to which the self is compromised by the loss of limbs can be calculated as the sum of the surface areas of all amputated parts. Literally counting on his body to bear out physiological laws, he finds that, having lost four-fifths of his original body weight, he adds up to no more than a "fraction of a man" (11). "The Case of George Dedlow" is in this sense a meditation on the impact of physical mutilation on manliness. If a man is "not a part, but the whole of his economy," to use Mitchell's words, what becomes of masculinity when parts of a man are missing? What, the story asks, does it mean to be a "fraction of a man"?

By stressing the centrality of the body to personhood, Mitchell's story expresses a set of concerns that pervaded Victorian ideas about embodiment in general, and dismemberment in particular, in both Britain and America. Simply put, amputation exposed, and ultimately interrogated, the importance of physical wholeness to Victorian conceptions of identity. In fragmenting the body, amputation fractured ideas about the self—what it is, where it comes from, where it is located, and whether, in the absence of a complete body, it can ever be completely present. Moreover, anxieties about amputation's effect on identity took on expressly gendered contours over the course of the nineteenth century. The vast majority of amputations done in Britain and America in those years were performed on injured soldiers and industrial workers. Their bodies were the source material for medicine's study of amputation, allowing doctors to sharpen their surgical skills and to study the effects of limb loss over time.[3] As such, the broad questions amputation raised about the relationship of physical stability to selfhood encoded more pointed anxieties about the place of the male body in determining men's gender identity.

Victorian ideals of health, particularly of male health, centered on the concept of physical wholeness: a strong, vigorous body was a primary signifier of manliness, at once testifying to the existence of a correspondingly strong spirit and providing that spirit with a vital means of material expression.[4] Dismemberment disrupted this physical economy. It unmanned amputees, producing neurological disorders that gave the fragmented male body—or parts of it, anyway—a distinctly feminine side. Thrashing, twitching, and suffering from phantom pains, stumps showed a deep-rooted propensity for theatrical malingering that rivaled that of the hysteric herself. And like the hysteric, the dismembered man seemed to speak a fraudulent body language. Phantom limbs were the fabrications of anatomies vitally invested in representing themselves as whole; they formed a sort of neurological narrative, a story told by somatic structures, and so raised the unsettling possibility that the material body could be profoundly inauthentic, that a loss of physical integrity could lead to a falsification of the self. Stump pathology thus suggested not only that masculinity was contingent on physical integrity—that a man was only as complete as his body—but also that an effeminate pain pattern could undercut the essence of a man, that an incomplete man was not a true one. Where amputation produced bodies that routinely misrepresented themselves (as partly female, as completely whole), prosthetics contained the aberrant signs of the dismembered body within a more totalizing—and tangible—form.

Prosthetics figured in the Victorian imagination as the closural movement of amputation, putting an end to the body's unsettling counter-
narrative by materially effacing it as such. More specifically, prosthetics
engineered a fiction of physical wholeness in the interest of recuperating the laboring male body, symbolically resolving the problem of fractional men simply by making them seem to disappear. Redefining essence in utilitarian terms, so that what a man was became synonymous
with what he could do, artificial limbs installed a functional model of
selfhood in place of a shattered ideal of wholeness. They fixed up fractions of men by making their bodies work.

This chapter concerns itself with the discourse of amputation that
arose between about 1851, when the first "modern" artificial limbs were
displayed at the Crystal Palace exhibition, and 1914, when World War I
radically altered the experience and social construction of bodily mutilation.[5] The period between the Great Exhibition and the First World
War saw both the rise of industrial modernity—in the shape of a global
mass market and a fully bureaucratized, state-administered imperialism—and the modernization of dismemberment, in the form of improved surgical techniques and new prosthetic technologies. With its
broad historical dimensions and its focus on symbolic continuities between Britain and America, this chapter aims to show how dismemberment became a kind of symbolic index of modernity in ways that
crossed national boundaries.[6] Together, amputation and prosthetics
formed an absolutely material economy of representation, opening up
and working out cultural tensions about what bodies could and should
be on bodies themselves. The discourse of dismemberment staged a
progression through gendered ontologies of the physical: as the amputee passed from the feminine world of nervous debility to the masculine world of inexhaustible machinery, an outdated essentialism was
displaced, physically and ideologically, by a state-of-the-art materialism. The pragmatic treatment of dismembered men thus became a
means of telling a more comprehensive story about the loss and recovery of manliness under industrial capitalism. Prosthetics mobilized a
new framework for masculinity, one that could accommodate the vulnerability of the body to injury by capitalizing on the increasing capacity of machines to imitate, and even improve on, human flesh.

The Victorian discourse of dismemberment manufactured a manhood that was specially equipped to meet the physical and ideological demands of modernity, and as such it has much to tell us about contemporary invocations of prosthesis as a radical mechanism of materialist self-transcendence. "Prosthesis" circulates in contemporary cultural studies as a metaphor for the peculiar intimacy between body and machine in the electronic age; it has become a celebratory catchword for the special liberations promised by technology, liberations founded on a logic of bodily distantiation in which problems of human agency can be sidestepped by imagining machines as fabulously capable supplements to a comparatively limited flesh. A central claim of this chapter is that prosthesis-as-metaphor has been severed from its conceptual and material roots in a distinctly Victorian symbolic economy, one that used actual prosthetics to model a highly idealized—and deeply problematic—interdependency between man and machine. In this chapter I seek to repair that breach, elaborating on the historical conditions under which modern prosthetics emerged—as a technology, and, increasingly, as a metaphor for man's relationship to technology—in order, finally, to sketch a preliminary genealogy of our present fascination with the notion that at the body-machine interface lies a "prosthetic territory," a frontier of potential resistance whose liberatory effects derive, paradoxically, from a strategic complicity with and dependence on machines.[7]

PHANTOMS

Throughout the nineteenth century the mortality rate for amputation was extremely high, ranging from around 75 percent for amputations done at the hip to about 25 percent for those done at the ankle.[8] Nevertheless, so many amputations were performed that in 1871 Mitchell estimated that at least fifteen thousand American men who had lost a limb during the Civil War were still living ("Phantom Limbs" 564). Likewise, the number of people who survived mutilation in industrial accidents grew exponentially over time, comprising an ever more substantial population in their own right. Amputation became an increasingly visible phenomenon as the century progressed. As with mastectomy, advances in surgical techniques and the development of anesthesia and antisepsis made surgical dismemberment into a much more viable medical option than it had been in the past; the result was not only that more amputations were performed than ever before, but also that people began to survive them with more regularity.[9] However, even as amputation was used with increasing success to save lives, as Mitchell's story suggests, it also challenged notions of what it meant to be alive in the first place by raising troubling questions about the relationship of identity to embodiment in life and in death. In Louisa May Alcott's *Hospital Sketches* (1863), for instance, a veteran double amputee doubts whether the integrity of his body will be restored in the afterlife: "What a scramble there'll be for arms and legs, when we old boys come out of our graves, on the Judgment Day: wonder if we shall get our own again? If we do my leg will have to tramp from Fredericksburg, my arm from here, I suppose, and meet my body, wherever it may be" (31).[10]

This amputee's picture of eternally scattered souls speaks to the fundamental anxiety of amputation, which bodied forth in such strange configurations that it made people wonder just what a man lost when he lost a limb. In his 1854 treatise *The Science and Art of Surgery*, for instance, John Erichsen explicitly associates pathologically constituted stumps with feminine susceptibility. Whereas simple stump pain occurs in even the "strongest and healthiest subjects, and is entirely dependent on local causes," more serious symptoms such as particularly intense pain and convulsive twitching are deeply gendered, and as such are signs of a more general nervous affection: "This form of painful stump arises from constitutional causes, and invariably occurs in females, more particularly in those of the hysterical temperament, and who are subject to neuralgic pains elsewhere. In these cases the general cutaneous sensibility of the stump is increased; it is often the seat of convulsive jerkings or twitchings, and the pain is of a more or less intermittent character, being increased under the influence of various emotional and constitutional causes. . . . No excision of the nerves of the stump or even amputation higher up is of any avail: the disease being constitutional, will certainly return in each successive stump, until at last the shoulder or the hip may be reached without any permanent benefit accruing to the patient" (87). The notion that stump pathology is not only feminine, but female, had far-reaching consequences for medical and social understandings of the male amputee, whose manhood was thereby implicated in an effeminate pain pattern. Altering the body in ways that were as psychically threatening as they were physically therapeutic, amputation raised the possibility that cutting off a man's limb could cut a man off from himself.

As Erichsen's example suggests, medical writing about amputation associates the loss of a limb with a proportionate loss of gender: the amputee's masculinity is weakened insofar as parts of him begin to feel like a woman. Mitchell's own work on amputation, for instance, finds in the stump a series of markedly feminine traits. Asserting that stumps present a physiology "so new and peculiar" that they must be understood as separate somatic entities, Mitchell devotes an entire chapter to what he calls "the neural maladies of stumps" in his *Injuries of Nerves and Their Consequences* (1872).[11] Essentially beings unto themselves, stumps play by such different physiological rules that they can be unstable even when their owners are not: "The amputation of limbs gives rise to certain functional conditions"; stumps are "liable to certain nervous disorders, which are often intractable" (342–44). If amputation enervates George Dedlow, reducing him to a "larval" state, it more commonly induces nervous frenzy in the affected part, driving that piece of the male body mad. Engendering an essentially effeminate sensitivity— the stump is a raw nerve—amputation robs a man of his anatomical equanimity when it robs him of his limb. Existing in a state of "unstable equilibrium," stumps are "ready to respond excessively and without regularity to every excitation" (*Injuries* 363). Stumps have exquisite "sensibilities"—even relatively "healthy" ones tend "to respond by pain or spasmodic movements to causes which do not disturb normal parts"—and as such, they are extremely susceptible to "the most horrible neuralgias and to certain curious, spasmodic maladies." A hard-core neurotic whose afflictions arise "from inflamed or hardened conditions of the divided nerves," the stump aches and twitches at the slightest change in atmospheric pressure and palpitates during the performance of basic bodily functions ("Phantom Limbs" 564–65).[12] Morbidly perverse, it even has a sick sense of humor—pain typically runs down a lost leg during urination (*Injuries* 346). Displaying classic hysterical stigmata, stumps suffer from hyper- and anesthesias; they can be paralyzed, and they can even throw fits. Spasmodic stumps, for example, exhibit a kind of choreiform clownism, what Mitchell calls "automatic gymnastics." These stumps are prone to "thresh about in a wild and meaningless fashion so as to excite for [their] owner attention wherever he goes." Like most malingerers, however, they can compose themselves when it suits them—one "politely showed an interest in its owner by ceasing to quiver for the whole day on which he had made an offer of marriage" ("Phantom Limbs" 565).[13]

For Mitchell, amputation engenders a sort of liminal lunacy; the insane remainder of surgical trauma, the stump is a nervous wreck. As such, his picture of amputation implicitly substantiates the claim of such Victorian doctors as Henry Maudsley that "the forms and habits of mutilated men approach those of women" (35). Describing the pathology of amputation in terms of a prototypical hysteria, Mitchell suggests that cutting up the male body absolutely fragments that body's masculinity; that opening up a man allows a madwoman—or at least a piece of one—to come out.[14] Apprehending limb loss as a loss of gender, Mitchell's formulation set the tone for subsequent characterizations of stump pathology. A 1918 monograph by G. Martin Huggins entitled *Amputation Stumps: Their Care and After-Treatment*, for example, absolutely echoes Mitchell's terms. Its chapter on "Painful and Tender Stumps" catalogs the "symptoms" of unhealthy stumps as "hyperaesthesia over extensive areas, twitching and jumping of the stump, and even epileptiform fits" (135). The chapter includes a section on paralytic stumps, and one on what Huggins calls "Jumpy Stumps." A jumpy stump is "a certain type of neurotic stump which jumps whenever the patient thinks of it and goes into violent clonic movements whenever the surgeon approaches to examine it." There are three types of jumpy stumps: ones whose movements have an organic basis in bulbous nerve endings; "neurotic" ones, which, like many nervous women, stop acting up if they are "firmly grasped by the hand"; and "neurasthenic" stumps, which are "difficult to handle" in themselves, and which come attached to a "patient . . . clamouring for an operation." As if individuals of different sexes were involved, such cases require two courses of treatment: "surgical rest for the stump"—the lady—and for the remaining man, "occupation for the mind" (149).[15]

In depicting pathological stumps as hysterical women, doctors drew on cultural understandings of sexual difference to stress the stump's otherness, its total departure from both male body and masculine self: what is especially disturbing about the pathology of amputation, in the accounts of Mitchell and others, is precisely that the stump seems not to belong to the person to whom it is attached. Rather than suggesting that amputation feminizes the amputee, then, both Huggins and Mitchell imagine that the amputated body suffers from a sort of split personality, a nervous disease in which the stump's shattered nerves act out in ways that erode the amputee's masculinity—he is less than a man insofar as his injured part behaves like an unstable woman. Ideas about a biologically based sexual difference informed this figuration, not in order to suggest that amputation turned men into women, but rather to register the extent to which amputation made men alien to themselves.[16] Portraying parts of the amputee's anatomy as feminine thus enabled medicine to formulate the impact of dismemberment in terms of a loss, rather than a change, of gender. Figuring a man's injured parts as a feminine entity provided doctors with a way to imagine the amputee as less than himself, of indicating that he was not all there.

The association of amputation with a disruption of gender norms was so strong in nineteenth-century thinking that metaphors of dismemberment could even function as a kind of shorthand for more overtly sexual kinds of loss. George Eliot, for instance, uses amputation as a figure for spiritual severance between a man and a woman, repeatedly describing men who lose their better halves as emotional cripples. In *Middlemarch* (1871–72), Fred Vincy declares that "I have never been without loving Mary [Garth]. If I had to give her up, it would be like beginning to live on wooden legs" (356). Lydgate teaches himself to accept his disappointment in his wife Rosamond by thinking of her as a nonentity who cannot be expected to give him the support he requires: "The first great disappointment has been borne: the tender devotedness and docile admiration of the ideal wife must be renounced, and life must be taken up on a lower stage of expectations, as it is by men who have lost their limbs" (450–51). And when Will Ladislaw contemplates life without Dorothea, Eliot tells us that "there was no more foretaste of enjoyment in the life before him than if his limbs had been lopped off and he was making his fresh start on crutches" (553). Similarly, in *Adam Bede* (1859), Hetty Sorrel cuts Adam off from his capacity to love when the weight of her indiscretions crushes his ideal image of her: "Love, he thought, could never be anything to him but a living memory—a limb lopped off, but not gone from consciousness" (461). Using amputation as a trope for a masculinity that is inherently incomplete without a feminine appendage, Eliot abstracts and inverts medical models of male amputation. Whereas in medical literature the amputee's sexuality is compromised by the physical proximity of his evidently feminine stump, in Eliot's fiction a man will always already be cut off from himself unless his identity becomes dependent on and fundamentally indistinguishable from a woman.

Such metaphoric treatments of gender relations as an inherently dismembered proposition find their clinical counterpart in medical depictions of stump pathology as a form of physiological misrepresentation. Revealing a feminine propensity to hysteria—or rather, revealing a hysterical tendency to imitate femininity—stump disorder constitutes a form of disorderly signification, a telling confusion of body and gender, personality and parts. As if to say that stumps can not only speak for themselves but are also more articulate than the people to whom they are attached, Mitchell gathers evidence from "ninety stumps and the statements of fourteen persons"; his subsequent analysis concentrates on what he calls "stump speech" ("Phantom Limbs" 565), which comprises a virtual lexicon of somatoform distress. Whereas the empty gestures of spasmodic stumps make up a kind of biological babble, phantom limb pain, in which the amputee retains an acute, often painful awareness of the absent limb as a distinct presence, constitutes a more pronounced pathology; indeed, as a neurological effort to give shape to an otherwise disorderly set of somatic signs, it constitutes a distinct narrative form.

Mitchell himself coined the term *phantom limb* in 1871. Writing for *Lippincott's Magazine of Popular Literature and Science*, Mitchell was the first to attempt an extended, scientific explanation of a phenomenon doctors had noted in passing for hundreds of years.[17] While the amputee's ability to sense the lost limb had hitherto been explained in a spiritual sense—Lord Nelson felt that his ability to sense his lost arm confirmed the existence of his eternal soul, and Descartes used the phenomenon to support his theory that the soul was seated in the mind—Mitchell makes an expressly medical claim for the meaning of the amputated body, accounting for its phenomenology in strictly secular, somatic terms.[18] Calling it a "sensorial delusion," Mitchell reads the phantom limb as the nonsensical projection of an unstable stump (*Injuries* 348). Like the Victorian spirit medium, whose ability to conjure ghosts was associated with both hysterical susceptibility and fraudulent representation, the neurotic stump raps, knocks, thrashes, and strains in order to make up a ghost that feels real but isn't really there.[19] Phantom limbs are the "spectral technologies" of a short-circuited nervous system, the automatic—or autonomic—writing of a sensorium determined to bring its departed member back to life.[20] Rather than providing a spiritually soothing, if physically painful, proof of the existence of one's soul, then, the phantom is a medical emergency, often obliging "the sufferer to submit to a second amputation. In one instance, six amputations were done on one leg without relief" ("Phantom Limbs" 565). An anatomical aberration, the phantom limb is so disturbing that it is sometimes necessary to try to cut it off.[21]

Despite his evident concern with excising—or exorcising—not only spiritualist accounts of phantom limbs but also the phantoms themselves, Mitchell conserves a spectral tone in the metaphoric language he uses to describe a strictly neurological state. "It has long been known to surgeons that when a limb has been cut off the sufferer does not lose the consciousness of its existence," Mitchell wrote; "A person in this condition is haunted, as it were, by a constant or inconstant fractional phantom of so much of himself as has been lopped away—an unseen ghost of the lost part" ("Phantom Limbs" 565). In the context of hard science, "phantom limb" is more than simply an explanatory analogy; indeed, it defines a distinct anatomy. In other words, it functions less as a way of narrating neurology and more as a way of indicating the nervous system's tendency to narrate itself. Inducing phantom limbs in his patients by applying electricity to their stumps, Mitchell proved that they are simply "sensory hallucinations," signs of the body's systematic effort to re-member itself (*Injuries* 348).[22] As such, Mitchell's formulation is perfectly consistent with materialist theories of memory, which argue that the faculty of recollection is wholly embodied. Henry Maudsley claims that "in every nerve-cell there is memory, and not only so, but there is memory in every organic element of the body" (25); while in *Mind and Body* Alexander Bain observes that the memory is only as good as the body it belongs in: "The memory rises and falls with the bodily condition" (9).

Mitchell's model projects these hypotheses into the phantom limb, imagining that the dismembered body memorializes itself through the spectralization of the severed part; that the pathology of amputation is one in which physiology responds phantasmatically to its own fragmentation. Amputation, as Mitchell describes it, ceases to be the occasion for spiritual confirmation and instead exposes the body's unsettling ability to imagine the missing limb back into place. The outgrowth of the nervous system's effort to make sense of the body's pain, the phantom limb is a sort of sensation fiction, a story the body tells itself about its position in space. Regarding the phantom almost as a somatic souvenir, the graphic record of the maimed body's better days—"We have realized here, in regard to common sensations, the fable which describes the retina as retaining after death the last picture which fell upon its living concavity" (*Injuries* 354)—Mitchell develops an essentially literary biology in which the open-ended body is seen as naturally predisposed to plot its own closure. For him, the phantom limb is not a medical metaphor so much as it is an objective description of how the fragmented body has already metaphorized itself. Recasting the issue of resurrection as a problem of reconstruction, Mitchell's phantom is a symbol of salvation only insofar as it represents the body's imaginative effort to salvage itself.

While lay accounts like Lord Nelson's read the phantom as a reassuring sign that when a limb cannot be present in body it will always be there in soul, Mitchell takes the phantom as an instance of wishful physiological thinking. The phantom limb continually disrupts the amputee's ability to adjust to his altered anatomy by fooling him into feeling what is not actually there. Mitchell notes that even after twenty or thirty years men are so deceived by the sensation that they act upon it, often to unhappy effect. He describes a man who believed he had struck another man with his lost hand, another who was thrown from his horse when he switched the reins to an absent grip, and still another who was so nauseated by the failure of his phantom fingers to pick up his fork that his appetite was spoiled for years. Even though the phantom regularly deceives the body, it never quite gets it together. "The spirit member is never complete," Mitchell writes. "The foot or hand are most distinctly felt, and then ankle or wrist. The parts between these and the knee or elbow, as the case may be, are seemingly indistinct or absent, and any missing parts yet higher up are totally unfelt. In some cases, half a hand is gone, and only a phantom finger or two remain somewhere in the air, with an utter abolition of every other portion of the arm."[23] Not being grounded in reality, the phantom limb lacks roots. It wanders much the way the womb wanders in archaic accounts of hysteria, sometimes losing so much length that it merges with the stump. "A patient describing this condition insisted that the stump felt far less distinctly present than the hand, which, for him, appeared to lie in the stump, save that the finger-ends projected beyond it" ("Phantom Limbs" 567). The desperate measure of a disrupted bodily economy, the phantom limb figures as a sort of ill-conceived mental prosthetic; if it represents a natural urge to reconstitute the dismembered body, it also dramatically advertises that body's complete incapacity to get its own constitution right. One of Mitchell's patients complained, "Every morning I have to learn anew that my leg is enriching a Virginia wheat crop or ornamenting some horrible museum." And another said, "If . . . I should say, I am more sure of the leg which ain't than of the one that are, I guess I should be about correct" ("Phantom Limbs" 566–67). In Mitchell's model, the loss of anatomical integrity turns the body into a pathological liar.

Representing the pathology of amputation as a problem of somatic signification, Mitchell describes the stump's neurological deficit as a failed narrative form, the sign of a disordered and incomplete effort to reconstruct a coherent, unitary physical structure. As such, he exemplifies the more general tendency of Victorian medicine to refract issues of physical integrity through a problematic of gender by depicting the delusional stump as an affront to the amputee's manhood. Pathological stumps compromise a man by contradicting him: they not only yield to a deeply rooted urge to act like women, but also purposefully attempt to deceive the amputee into thinking he is still a whole man. For Mitchell, framing stump pathology as a form of hysterical malingering is thus not only a way of talking about amputation as a loss of manhood in an economy of difference that had difficulty conceiving of sexuality in anything other than binary terms, but also of figuring the mutilated male body as a failed representational system. According to Victorian medicine, most neuroses were on some level imaginary, the fictional productions of functional disorder. By contrast, the neural maladies of stumps functioned to produce the fiction of a natural order—they represented the body to itself as that which was not being represented at all. At once absolutely organic and utterly unreal—a lie told by a nervous lesion—phantom limb pain confounded body and image, and in the process reduced the amputee's masculinity to a mere figure of his stump's erroneous speech.

Despite ample opportunities for scientific observation in "civil life" and "asylums for soldiers," amputation was an ontological conundrum, a profoundly difficult phenomenon to apprehend. Neither the amputee nor those around him can be depended on for an accurate account of "the physiological conditions which arise in persons who have been so unhappy as to lose limbs," Mitchell notes. Exuding an absolutely infectious illogic, the pathology of amputation spreads beyond the space of the dismembered body to deprive even intact individuals of all sense of proportion: "The natural tendency of many witnesses, especially among the uneducated, is to color too strongly their answers in regard to points which excite wonder or sympathy" ("Phantom Limbs" 564). The functional illiteracy of the disarticulated body, in which attempts at self-inscription express only a gross incompetence, authorizes a more general categorical confusion; amputation confounds figures so completely that it becomes impossible to tell a truncated body from a tall tale.

"The Case of George Dedlow," for instance, was taken for a true story by the American public even though it was framed in openly fictional terms. Serving as a vehicle for describing the impact of amputation on identity in less clear-cut cases, Dedlow's limbless body functions as the fictional exception that proves the factual rule. He is himself a statistical impossibility—"so far as we are aware, no one survived the removal of all four limbs above the elbows and knees, although such a case is said to have occurred in the Napoleonic Wars"—and while a certain amount of expertise might be necessary to identify the "useless torso" as a textual trope, the grotesque nature of the tale's final physical tableau should clarify its generic status ("Phantom Limbs" 564; "George Dedlow" 5). While at a séance, Dedlow is visited by the spirits of his lost legs. Identifying themselves by rapping out their specimen numbers—"UNITED STATES ARMY MEDICAL MUSEUM, Nos. 3486, 3487"—the legs attach themselves to Dedlow's stumps and temporarily restore his ability to walk: "A strange wonder filled me, and, to the amazement of every one, I arose, and, staggering a little, walked across the room on limbs invisible to them or me. . . . [I]t was no wonder I staggered, for, as I briefly reflected, my legs had been nine months in the strongest alcohol" (11). As flexible as Dedlow's pickled parts, Mitchell's narrative bows to the dreamwork of phantom limbs, allowing them to materialize as prosthetic extensions of the self, and then sliding out from under its own (admittedly flimsy) symbolic recovery. As if to say that the only real spiritual solution for missing limbs is the one that preserves them in bottles, both Dedlow and the difficulty he embodies end up stumped: "I felt myself sinking slowly. My legs were going, and in a moment I was resting feebly on my two stumps upon the floor. It was too much. All that was left of me fainted and rolled over senseless" (11). Steeping his story in contradiction, Mitchell leaves any claim to realism without a leg to stand on.[24]

Even as the story openly encourages disbelief by putting an improbable character through a series of increasingly impossible paces, "Many persons . . . accepted it as true. Inquiries were made as to the whereabouts of the sufferer, and in an interior county of New York a subscription was actually started for the unhappy victim" ("Phantom Limbs" 564); indeed, "benevolent persons went to the 'Stump Hospital,' in Philadelphia, to see the sufferer and to offer him aid" (Introduction ix). Mitchell was deeply alarmed by the gullibility of an audience that had mistaken an obviously sensational fiction for an objective statement of fact, explaining that he had simply taken "advantage of the freedom accorded a writer of fiction" to describe "as belonging to this class of sufferers certain psychological states so astounding in their character that he certainly could never have conceived it possible that his humorous sketch, with its absurd conclusion, would for a moment mislead any one" ("Phantom Limbs" 564). It was precisely the least believable aspects of the narrative, however, that played most strongly on public sensibilities: "The spiritual incident at the end of the story," for instance, "was received with joy by the spiritualists as a valuable proof of the truth of their beliefs" (Introduction ix). Recognizing that his narrative had induced a kind of public neurosis, Mitchell rewrote his description of amputation in "Phantom Limbs," hoping that by confining himself to facts, he could reconfigure public perception along more reasonable lines: "The present description of what the amputated really feel and suffer may possibly serve to correct such erroneous beliefs." Imagining that by choosing "cases for observation with great care" he can limit the uncertain significance of mutilated anatomy (as if some figurations were more authentic than others), Mitchell insists on reinstating the distinctions his subject has already irrevocably broken down (564). Even so, the amputated body disallows detached observation; its "pathological peculiarities" (Watson 353) generate a kind of sympathetic separation anxiety in its witnesses, leaving them as disoriented as it is.

The public reaction to "The Case of George Dedlow" points to a central epistemological difficulty posed by dismemberment. Even the most faithful renderings of amputation play tricks on the eye, so that pictures of incompletion always look like flawed or incomplete pictures (fig. 6), and diagrams confuse the difference between bodies so thoroughly that they do more to depict a crisis of representation than they do to delimit proper surgical technique. In figure 7, for instance, nineteen fingers surround the one being removed, as if to insist that with so many digits around, one will never be missed; in figure 8 the doctor's body is cut off—the patient's arm is being amputated by amputated arms. As these drawings suggest, the dismembered body is so far removed from standard frames of reference that it cannot measure up to even the most realistic expectations. Creating a kind of "mass confusion," amputation is so unconventional that it is all but impossible to represent it at all (fig. 9).

MECHANISM

Appending a literature of reconstruction to the discourse of dismemberment much as prosthetics themselves were appended to the dismembered body, Victorians situated the prosthetic reassembly of the body as the natural end point of amputation. Artificial limbs were the answer to the amputated body's wayward signs, stabilizing both its chaotic symptoms and its capacity to confuse by lifting the amputee into a new (and implicitly improved) technology of self. Prosthetics

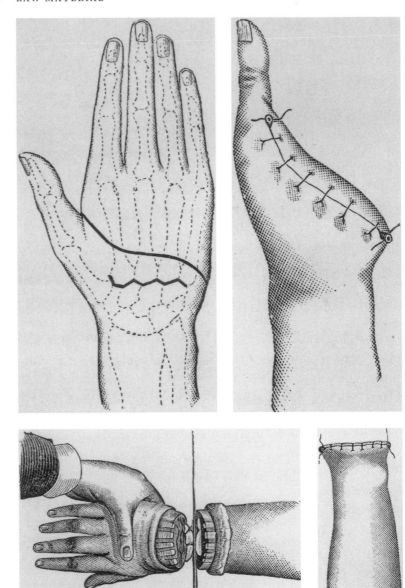

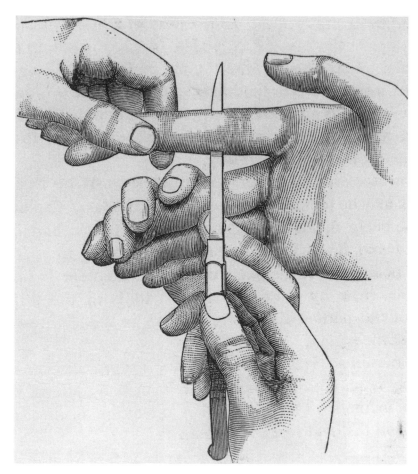

Fig. 6. (opposite) Pictures of incompletion. From B. A. Watson, *Treatise on Amputation of the Extremities and Their Complications* (1885). Courtesy of the College of Physicians, Philadelphia.

Fig. 7. (above) Excessive fingers. From B. A. Watson, *Treatise on Amputation of the Extremities and Their Complications* (1885). Courtesy of the College of Physicians, Philadelphia.

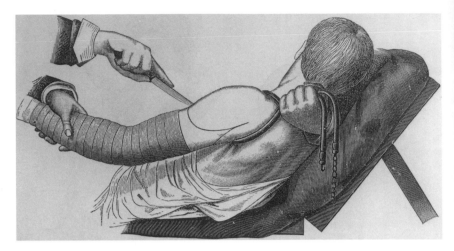

Fig. 8. Amputated arms amputating. From B. A. Watson, *Treatise on Amputation of the Extremities and Their Complications* (1885). Courtesy of the College of Physicians, Philadelphia.

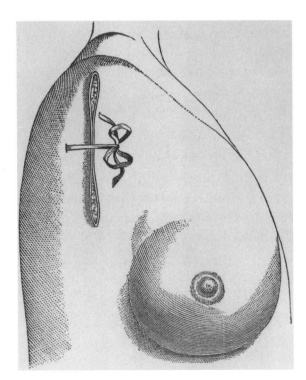

Fig. 9.
Nonsensical torso.
From B. A.
Watson, *Treatise on Amputation of the Extremities and Their Complications* (1885). Courtesy of the College of Physicians, Philadelphia.

supplied the stump with a much-needed form of closure (as if to finish the tragic fragment with a happy ending), working within the categorical constraints of the amputated body by reading it back at itself. Capable of constructing the fragmented body as essentially whole—of narrating it as not being narrated at all—the artificial limb stands as an absolutely material form of fiction making, a means of restoring the integrity of the self by passing off a made-up anatomy as real. Turning on a fundamental incongruity between two conceptual systems by defining them as the same, prosthetics cobble together a utilitarian imperative and a narrative impulse, so that the fact of getting a man back on his feet effectively mobilizes a fiction of his physical wholeness for the observer (who can't detect them), and even for the wearer himself (who can forget them). As a man with two artificial legs wrote to A. A. Marks, one of the premier limb makers during the latter half of the nineteenth century, "Your labors have restored me to my feet, and I am, for all practical purposes, myself again" (*Patent* 197).

Artificial limbs reconstitute the amputated body by breaking down operative distinctions between human flesh and other material forms. Suggesting that building up the body simply reverses the damage done by taking it apart, the discourse of prosthesis positions the artificial limb as the structural inversion of amputation even as it involves a complete change of terms (prosthetics necessarily operate on a principle of substitution). As such, prosthesis contains the pathologically signifying body of the amputee in a conceptual structure that drastically limits the kinds of stories it can tell. By locking "fractions of men" in a logic that strategically fails to register certain material and conceptual forms of difference, prosthesis claims to restore men to themselves by merging their bodies with machines. Compensating a man by supplying him with copies of himself, prosthesis contends that nature can be made through mechanization—in other words, that essence can be re-created through imitation, and that identity is something that can be attached.

Moreover, the slippages between body and object, man and machine, nature and culture that are central to the discourse of prosthesis have a "natural" basis in the physiology of prosthesis itself. Simply conceptual manifestations of an absolutely material process, the gaps in the logic of prosthesis cannot quite be identified as gaps at all—the basic premise of prosthesis, that masculinity can be restored by defining away the difference between body and machine, is indistinguishable from its physiology: the amputee recovers his inner coherence only after his body has been elided with an object outside itself. Both Weir Mitchell and William James observed that phantom limbs tended to fuse with artificial ones; providing an acceptable space for the body's excess sensation, the artificial limb becomes the repository for the stump's residual feelings. As errant as they are when their stumps are unattached, then, phantoms typically assume the position of the prosthesis as soon as it is applied: "Generally the position of the lost leg follows that of the stump and artificial leg. If one is flexed the other seems flexed; if one is extended so is the other; if one swings in walking the other swings with it" (James 3).[25] According to James, the phantom limb is a "projection" that collapses "fancy" into "feeling": "I have seldom seen a more plausible lot of evidence for the view that imagination and sensation are but differences of vividness in an identical process" (8). Absolutely amenable to the power of suggestion (the "lost foot . . . sympathizes sometimes with the foot which remains. If one is cold, the other feels cold. One man writes that whenever he walks through puddles and wets his sound foot, his lost foot feels wet too" [James 11]), the phantom almost automatically follows the example of the artificial limb.[26] Moreover, artificial limbs depend on phantoms even as they discipline them— prosthetics simply don't work unless phantom limbs fill them up. Containing the very force that animates them, artificial limbs work by foreclosing on the inarticulate expressions of amputated anatomy. Sealing off the transgressive potential of the stump by straitening its spasms and even silencing its speech, they supply the amputated body with a material means of making sense. Imagining that the artificial limb can confine the stump to sensible conversation (in more ways than one, prosthetics might be said to shut the stump up), James and Mitchell make explicit what the discourse of amputation more generally implies, that a lost disposition can be re-created by splicing a mechanical member to the remains of a man. Moving from a literary biology to a functional technology—from a degenerative physical condition to a productive social position—prosthetics remakes the essential self by way of a kind of biomechanical bricolage: phantom limbs talk the talk that enables artificial ones to walk the walk.[27]

The premise that self-contained individuals can be made up from man-made materials thus finds its physical complement in the artificial limb's ability to realize the dismembered body's insubstantial effort to complete itself—if phantom limbs signify a break in the body's logic, artificial ones stand for the possibility of both anatomical and epistemological repair. Setting in motion an anatomy whose inner coherence derives from elision with an outside object, artificial limbs brace up the body's own reconstructive impulse by fusing the body and its substitute in a single structure of representation. In so doing, prosthetics literalize Foucault's notion of a "discursive orthopedics," the mechanism by which Victorians produced bodies that seemed naturally to voice the truth of their sexuality (*History of Sexuality* 29). Foucault writes that during the eighteenth century the middle class believed "itself obliged to amputate from its body a sex that was useless, expensive, and dangerous as soon as it was no longer given over exclusively to reproduction"; by contrast, nineteenth-century culture was oriented toward providing this disembodied middle class with "a body to be cared for, protected, cultivated, and preserved . . . by equipping itself with— among other resources—a technology of sex" (123). Moreover, Foucault imagines this new technology of sex to be itself a prosthetic entity, a mechanism for managing the "juncture" between "body" and "population": sex is "implanted" in the Victorian body as that body is in turn "implanted in reality" (147, 29, 72). Artificial limbs "implant" an otherwise dislocated amputee in "reality"—home, street, market, work—by supplying him with a functional technology of manhood, a support system whose levers, cogs, pulleys, and springs operate, paradoxically, to sustain the fiction of a unified, integrated self.

Prosthetics allay anxieties about dismemberment by describing the dissolution of bodily boundaries as their recovery and imagining that anatomical integrity can be restored by way of bodily distantiation. They mobilize a logic of disjunction, a mechanism by which disparate parts can be combined into unified wholes, and self and other can be defined as the same. Mechanizing the amputee in order to naturalize him, the discourse of prosthesis redistributes the qualities of personhood across an economy of body and machine. As if to say that as long as you can move around, it doesn't matter how you do it, prosthetics focus on the final product to the exclusion of origins; as far as they are concerned, the end obfuscates the means: "making [the] maimed whole" by effecting the "removal of . . . disabilities *for all practical purposes,*" the discourse of artificial limbs asserts that, in order to recover his essential self, a man need only be technically complete (quoted in Marks, *Treatise on Artificial Limbs* 397, 317; emphasis added). As ontologically unstable as they are structurally sound, prosthetics piece individual bodies together even as they take the idea of the body itself apart. Sidestepping questions of individual essence by changing the subject, artificial limbs remasculinize the amputee by shifting the focus from his inner qualities to what he can actually do.

Artificial limbs thus provided a solid vehicle for a humanist politics of self-realization, modeling a physiology of compliance in which bodily recovery became synonymous with social recuperation. Defining essence in terms of what a body can do instead of what a body is—or rather, by defining what the body does *as* what it is—prosthetics set in motion a kind of utilitarian essentialism, a working model of selfhood that assumes identity is only ever what you make of it. Where amputation undercuts the amputee's masculinity by producing a feminine space within the male body, for instance, prosthetics assert that the dismembered body can cease to differ from itself if it simply makes a reasonable effort to do so. Treating the stump as a purely technical difficulty, prosthetics convert the hysterical appendage into a useful member simply by putting it to work. Limb makers and surgeons agreed that the stump could be kept in line only if it was routinely subjected to the disciplinary action of the artificial limb. Arguing that the amputee should be fitted as soon as possible after surgery to prevent an otherwise inevitable decline, limb maker J. F. Rowley insisted that "if you would have your stump leg strong, then as early as conditions permit, you must put it into training. . . . [T]here is nothing which will discipline and strengthen a stump leg as effectually as an artificial leg properly applied and carefully used" (72). If left to its own devices, the stump rapidly degenerates into a helpless invalid. Marks was certain that "delay in applying an artificial limb gives the stump an opportunity to become enervated from disuse, soft, flabby, and large from lack of exercise." "The muscles of an amputated limb not only become undisciplined," one physician said, "but they also become atrophied, shrunken, and effeminate, and the longer they are unused the more atrophied they become. . . . [I]nstead of a hard and firm stump, [the amputated limb] has more the appearance of a mass of quivering jelly" (quoted in Marks, *Treatise* 310).[28]

Artificial limbs circumvent such sexual regression, making a "hard and firm" member out of the helpless dependent by means of a rigorous form of occupational therapy. If "a stump, before it is called upon to operate an artificial limb is an inactive remnant of an active member of the body," that same stump quickly becomes an old hand at running its mechanical attachment; indeed, it becomes a skilled machinist in its own right (Marks, *Treatise* 321). Like the laborer himself, the stump is tempered by its occupation, stabilized by constant use: "The hands of a laborer are strong and hard because he uses them in performing his work. The hands of a person not accustomed to manual labor are soft, tender, and delicate and become easily blistered, simply because they have not been disciplined. The same principle is applicable to stumps" (309). The undisciplined stump may be a kind of hysterical woman, a volatile appendage dragging the amputee down, but the ideal stump is a working stiff, a man of steady habits who has been taught to know his place. Working out anxieties about a lost integrity by treating the body as a cultural construct—the stump is, after all, a product of its environment—artificial limbs restore the amputee's inner coherence by situating him in a new frame of reference. Treating amputation as a problem of unemployment, prosthetics rehabilitate recalcitrant physiologies by professionalizing them; as such, they stand for the transformative power of work itself. Blurring the distinction between effort and essence in order to model a harmonious and mutually beneficial relationship between man and machine, prosthetics enable a perfectly integrated and humane relationship between work and product to be imagined. As a machine that cannot be detached from the labor that makes it seem to come alive, prosthetics model a kinder, gentler capitalism—or at least one that can mystify the conditions of its possibility by casting power relations as perfect symbiosis. Depicting the product of labor as a blithely laboring self, prosthetics encode a utopian fantasy of industry in which factory work consolidates the worker's individuality instead of taking it away.[29]

The means by which the stump is brought in line with the rest of the body thus captures the process by which that body ultimately recovers its social standing—putting the stump to work recuperates the amputee's masculinity by making his stump conform to the rest of his body, just as making the amputee's body work resituates him in the social sphere by allowing him to fit in, physically and professionally, with other men of his class. Firmly locating the identity of the amputee in his ability to perform physically demanding tasks, artificial limbs articulate a sort of functionalist work ethic—all the amputee needs to be essentially himself is a working body. Treating the loss of a limb as a loss of motion, and demonstrating the power of the artificial limb to restore physical capability, the discourse of prosthesis defines masculinity as mobility—prosthetics make a "new man" out of the amputee by enabling him to do what he did before. Tricked out with an artificial limb, "not a soul has . . . occasion to suspect his actual make-up" because "his movements are graceful, his appearance is natural, his step is firm and elastic" (quoted in Marks, *Patent* 162). Indeed, the discourse of prosthesis routinely supports the assertion that the artificial limb "has made a new man of me" with a list of what the limb enables the new man to do: "My leg is amputated four inches below the body," wrote a wearer of one of Marks's legs with rubber feet. "I do considerable hard work, can carry 125 pounds on my shoulder, get on or off a train going eight miles an hour, ride horseback, get thrown off occasionally, and am not in constant dread of breaking my leg as I have seen wearers of other legs" (209).[30] So it is that when the amputee recovers his full range of motion, the "sense of loss is reduced to a minimum," and he can even forget the artificiality of the limb itself: "I have become so accustomed to [my artificial leg] that it has become a part of me" (149, 232). The integrity of the body is recovered when its "power is complete" (Marks, *Treatise* 135). While the amputated body never quite makes sense, that of the rebuilt man speaks for itself. Able to walk, run, jump, ride, climb, lift, and even skate with ease, he is "art practically exemplified," poetry in motion (Marks, *Patent* 149) (figs. 10–15).

With its emphatic focus on the relationship between context and recovery, and its equation of masculinity with mobility, then, the discourse of prosthesis consistently links bodily condition to social position. Indeed, the discourse indicates that in moving around, the

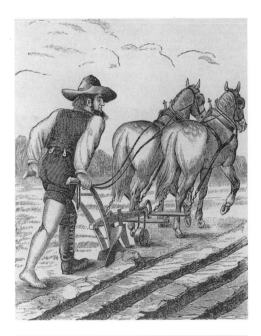

Fig. 10. Prosthetic ploughman. From A. A. Marks, *Treatise on Marks' Patent Artificial Limbs with Rubber Hands and Feet* (1888). Courtesy of the College of Physicians, Philadelphia.

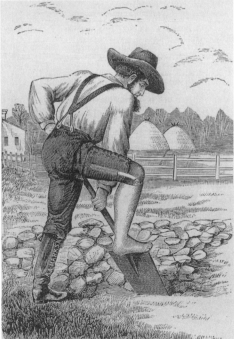

Fig. 11. Prosthetic digger. From A. A. Marks, *Treatise on Marks' Patent Artificial Limbs with Rubber Hands and Feet* (1888). Courtesy of the College of Physicians, Philadelphia.

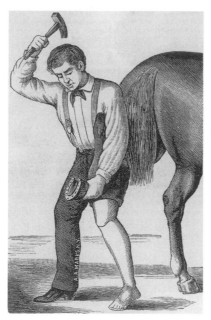

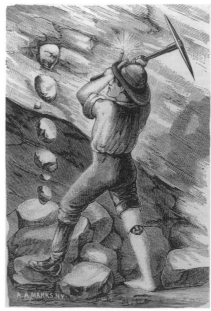

Fig. 12. Prosthetic farrier. From
A. A. Marks, *Treatise on Marks'*
Patent Artificial Limbs with Rubber
Hands and Feet (1888). Courtesy of
the College of Physicians,
Philadelphia.

Fig. 13. Prosthetic miner. From
A. A. Marks, *Treatise on Marks'*
Patent Artificial Limbs with Rubber
Hands and Feet (1888). Courtesy of
the College of Physicians,
Philadelphia.

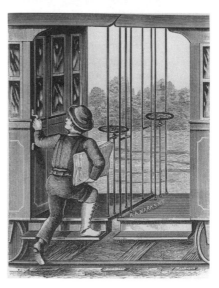

Fig. 14. Man leaping on artificial
leg. From A. A. Marks, *Treatise on*
Marks' Patent Artificial Limbs with
Rubber Hands and Feet (1888).
Courtesy of the College of
Physicians, Philadelphia.

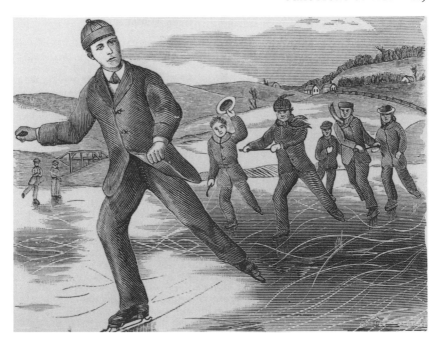

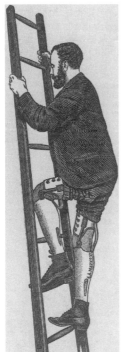

Fig. 15. Ice skater with artificial leg. From A. A. Marks, *Treatise on Marks' Patent Artificial Limbs with Rubber Hands and Feet* (1888). Courtesy of the College of Physicians, Philadelphia.

Fig. 16. Climbing the evolutionary ladder. From A. A. Marks, *Treatise on Marks' Patent Artificial Limbs with Rubber Hands and Feet* (1888). Courtesy of the College of Physicians, Philadelphia.

amputee is always on some level moving up. As we have already seen, artificial limbs make it possible for the amputee to climb a few rungs on the evolutionary ladder (a "first-class fit" [Marks, *Patent* 357] not only effects a sort of localized sex change, but, more fundamentally, raises the amputee from the "larval state" of a George Dedlow to the impressive stature of a physically cultured man). They also prevent the amputee from sliding down the social scale (fig. 16). While artificial limbs only ever allow the amputee to maintain the position he held before his loss, the ability to work at all is perceived as a marked improvement in his condition. As *Appleton's Journal* marveled in 1875, "Think of supporting a large family on an artificial leg, and dandling a baby on an artificial knee!" (Rideing 783). Artificial limbs thus instantiate a peculiarly static model of personal advancement—the rebuilt man is only ever running to stand still. Indeed, simply maintaining his station in the world involves him in an ongoing competition with physically perfect men—as one wearer somewhat defensively insisted, "I have been so thoroughly restored by your patent that really I cannot see or feel that I am different to persons in possession of their natural limbs. I do not take a second place to anybody" (Marks, *Patent* 310).

The discourse of prosthesis is thus infused with class consciousness, suggesting that a man cannot occupy a meaningful social position unless he is physically complete. Examples of this conflation of physical and social mobility abound in Victorian writing about amputation. In Dickens's *Our Mutual Friend* (1864–65), the one-legged ballad seller Silas Wegg goes to great lengths to recover the bone from his amputated leg because he is convinced that he cannot be a successful social climber without it: "I have a prospect of getting on in life and elevating myself by my own independent exertions . . . and I shouldn't like—I tell you openly I should *not* like—under such circumstances, to be what I may call dispersed, a part of me here, and a part of me there, but should wish to collect myself like a genteel person" (82). Likewise, in Trollope's *He Knew He Was Right* (1869), a postman with an old-fashioned wooden leg is categorically dismissed: "There is a general understanding that the wooden-legged men in country parishes should be employed as postmen, owing to the great steadiness of demeanour which a wooden leg is generally found to produce. It may be that such men are slower in their operations than would be bi-ped postmen; but as all private employers of labour demand labourers with two legs, it is well that the lame and halt should find a refuge in the less exacting service of the government" (167). Working about as smoothly as the postal system itself, the mailman's body may be good enough for government work, but it is not much good for anything else.

Trollope's model of the limb that makes the wearer over in its own image is a recurrent theme in nineteenth-century figurations of prosthetics, which see artificial limbs as a socially significant problem of synecdoche. Imagining that parts invariably take over the wholes they are reconstituting, authors such as Trollope and Dickens suggest that wearing artificial limbs—particularly limbs of lesser make—undermines the amputee's claim to humanity by making him vulnerable to a kind of infiltration, or contamination, from below. In *Our Mutual Friend,* for instance, Silas Wegg's quest to recover the bone of his amputated leg is made all the more urgent by the fact that its replacement is spreading to the rest of his body—"he was so wooden a man that he seemed to have taken his wooden leg naturally, and rather suggested to the fanciful observer, that he might be expected—if his development received no untimely check—to be completely set up with a pair of wooden legs in about six months" (46). Similarly, in *Pickwick Papers* (1836–37) wooden legs demonstrate both moral deterioration and subsequent reform. A one-legged teetotaler testifies that he "Used to wear second-hand wooden legs and drink a glass of hot gin and water regularly every night—sometimes two. . . . Found the second-hand wooden legs split and rot very quickly; is firmly persuaded that their constitution was undermined by the gin and water. . . . Buys new wooden legs now and drinks nothing but water and weak tea. The new legs last twice as long as the others used to do, and he attributes this solely to his temperate habits" (505). Although here Dickens depicts the moral degeneration of the alcoholic amputee as a process that can be both aided and arrested by the quality of his limbs, he nevertheless maintains the assumption that the amputee is in some very material sense the property of his own prosthesis. As if to suggest that as marginal members of society they are always already dead wood, Dickens represents the poor as particularly prone to this kind of physical appropriation.

As these examples suggest, the rhetorical construction of masculinity as mobility and the related premise that prosthetics restore the amputee's humanity by enabling him to work exist alongside a deep-seated anxiety that reconstructing men really only mechanizes them, and that artificial limbs finally dehumanize the subjects they are used to restore. Indeed, anxieties and optimisms about prosthetics are so similar that they frequently slide imperceptibly into one another. Edgar Allan Poe's 1839 story, "The Man That Was Used Up," for instance, celebrates the constitutive powers of prosthetics as a means of taking them to task. Centering on a man who has more artificial parts than authentic ones, Poe's story critiques the logic of prosthesis by turning it inside out. Having lost the bulk of his body in battle, Brevet Brigadier General John A. B. C. Smith represents an extreme of physical mutilation. Minus his limbs, shoulders, scalp, and an eye; toothless, tongueless, and without a palate; he is unspeakably disarticulated, a "nondescript" (270). Strategically substituting mechanical parts for the ones he has lost, "the man that was used up" compensates for his physical deficiencies through an elaborate ritual of replacement; he daily effects what the narrator calls an "inexplicable evolution" from an inhuman "it," "an exceedingly odd looking bundle of something" (269–70), into a "truly fine-looking fellow," a man whose artificial anatomy strikes the unsuspecting observer as a "remarkable" assemblage of the finest natural endowments (259). A veritable pattern of Victorian manhood, the officer figures as the ultimate man of parts.

Asking what it means for the self to become essentially supplemental—for a man to become his own body double—Poe's story sees prosthetics as a problem of individual constitution. A product of what he calls "the rapid march of mechanical invention," the officer's very speech patterns echo the rhythms of his automated anatomy. As if the mechanization of his body had made over his mind, his language is as jerky as his movements, and his metaphors are as mixed as he is: "I say, the most *useful*—the most truly *useful* mechanical contrivances, are daily springing up like mushrooms, if I may so express myself, or, more figuratively, like—ah—grasshoppers—like grasshoppers . . . about us and ah—ah—ah—around us!" (263). A man who has no identity apart from his apparatus, his autonomy is automatonic: a "gentleman of . . . undoubted dimension," he carries himself with "rectangular precision" and enjoys all the "dignity of colossal proportion" (261). In Poe's story, the prosthetic self has been made over by its additions; by definition (and by design) a cultural construct, the officer's *"remarkable . . .* something" is a ready-made phenomenon, a patent imitation for the real thing (261). Supplemented within an inch of his life, the general is finally little more than an elaborate put-on. Imagining that artificial limbs stage a sort of corporeal takeover, Poe depicts prosthetics as the occasion of an anatomical inversion in which body becomes copy and substitute gains substance.

Animated by the fundamental paradox of prosthetics—that the dismembered body cannot be rearticulated without also being objectified—Poe's story can be read as a macabre vision of industrial culture, a hysterical image of the displacement of body by machine. By the end of the story, the tenuous balance between the two has degenerated into a complete insanity of parts—as we watch the officer assemble himself in the story's final scene, we learn that he has parts for organs that can't be replaced (he speaks with a synthetic palate), and parts for organs that can't actually be removed (he wears a prosthetic chest); that he retains the properties of limbs in the absence of the limbs themselves (we see him screw on a leg even though he hasn't any arms), and that some of his artificial parts actually work (he sees better out of his glass eye than his real one).[31]

Where Poe imagines that the blurring of the boundary between body and object winds up compromising the amputee's humanity—in "The Man That Was Used Up," prosthetics only make a man less coherent than he was before—limb makers in the latter half of the century argued that state-of-the-art limbs could reconstitute shattered natures by mystifying their own mechanical qualities. An article published in *Appleton's Journal* in 1875 explicitly articulates this recuperative fantasy. Entitled "Patched-up Humanity," the essay praises "the dexterity of artisans in human-repair shops" for their role in remaking mutilated men, imagining the body as an assemblage of parts which, when broken, can be fixed up almost as good as new: "Such improvements have been made in late years . . . that, in all but sense of touch, an artificial leg performs the most important duties of a natural one, allowing the wearer to walk, run, or sit with ease, and to endure an astonishing degree of fatigue in an upright position" (Rideing 783–84). Standing as the quintessential triumph of industrial culture—in 1895 *Scientific American* ranked the limb maker with the surgeon "in the good he does to humanity," adding that "it would be hard to find a more beneficent example of the progress of mechanical science than that afforded by the peculiar industry" of prosthesis—the artificial limb reduces amputation to a minor inconvenience: it is "not as serious as the impairment of health or the loss of any one of the senses" ("Improved Artificial Limbs" 52). Although the "implements of civilization" have had a "distressing effect in dismembering the human body," they make up for it by effectively "removing the disabilities of the cripple" (Marks, *Treatise* 17, 22): "Science and the industrial arts present no higher evidence of progress than that observable in the perfection of surgical appliances designed to replace portions of the human form removed by innumerable causes" (Marks, *Patent* 148). For Marks, prosthetics and progress are effective indexes of one another: industrialization is principally to blame for dismemberment, but it redeems itself by undoing the tragedy of loss as such. Able to reproduce the body as mechanism, to make nature by design, artificial limbs ostensibly stand as the ultimate instance of "progress." As capable of conferring naturalness as they are of taking it away, they are—almost—living proof of liberal ideals.

Ironically, then, artificial limbs worked to rationalize laissez-faire attitudes toward progress at precisely the point where those attitudes would seem to be least tenable: the mutilated male body. Fixed up nearly as good as new by the same system that crippled him, the prosthetic man became a symbol of all that was possible in the modern world of manufacture, a walking advertisement for the personal and social benefits to be had from a full-scale embrace of machine culture. Proposing objectification as a viable strategy of selfhood, prosthetics were symbols of freedom—to move in the world, to advance through hard work, and even, increasingly, to leave the body behind. Asserting that "for all practical purposes" the amputee could absolutely recover his losses (albeit on the installment plan), prosthetics undercut the notion of the body as irreducible and put a model of anatomy as infinitely reproducible in its place. As A. A. Marks wrote, "What has been done can be done again" (*Treatise* iv). Indeed, the guiding impulse behind the technological development of artificial limbs was the idea that in reassembling the body, prosthetics could be made to resemble the flesh they were replacing. Limbs made over the latter half of the nineteenth century, with their rubber feet and hands, custom-fitted

wood-and-wax sockets, ball-bearing joints, and self-correcting sus-
penders, represented a marked improvement over older makes, which
were "so imperfect that no one was deceived by them." Old-fashioned
limbs seemed to bear out Poe's model of prosthetics, mechanizing the
amputee without actually fixing him up—with their "movable, clattering ankle-joints," the wearer was constantly in danger of breaking
down: "His entrance into a parlor was mistaken for the complaint of a
broken-down chair, or the squeak of a rat. When he moved in the
street, people turned round, expecting to see a wheelbarrow in want of
grease approaching, and when—awful moment!—he cast himself on his
knees before his adored one, his impassioned utterances were accompanied with rattling noises which suggested the unrest of a fallen spirit
in torment" (Rideing 783). "Only rattle-traps at the best" (Marks, *Patent* 245), wooden limbs "betrayed the wearer at every step" (Rideing
783). By contrast, newer models concealed their mechanical compo-
nents; only by looking inside them could the "combination of ugly iron
bolts, rods, and screws, which give the thing its movements" be dis-
cerned. As the century progressed, technological innovation allowed
the appearance of physical trauma to be silently corrected—the modern
artificial limb "is noiseless, and only an expert can detect it" (Rideing
783). Less mechanical because they were more advanced, the new limbs
blended with the body so naturally that they were more like family
members than they were like machines: "The foot which you have
supplied me has done its duty nobly. It clings to me with the stern
affection of a parent, never slips, always responds to the movement of
the ankle, and generally behaves as if it were acquainted with me inti-
mately since my birth," wrote one wearer. Another proclaimed, "My
leg is my best friend; it is what I love the most, and without it my life
would be miserable" (Marks, *Patent* 161, 254).

The best artificial limbs "counterfeited" the look and feel of flesh so
perfectly that people could be fooled into thinking they were the genuine article.[32] Endorsing an ethics of deception, advertisers argued that
the only way for the amputee to be true to himself was to lie to every-
body else. J. F. Rowley told potential customers, "One of your reasons
for buying an artificial leg is to disguise or hide your loss from the public;
you want to appear as a man, and you can do this only by learning to use
the leg perfectly. . . . The man who hitches, limps, or swings while

walking, deceives no one, for all know he has an artificial leg" (84). Even as the logic of prosthetics posits an implicit priority of body over thing, presuming not only that the body is ultimately inimitable (by definition a substitute just isn't the same) but also that the original absolutely differs, in quantity and in kind, from its replacement (it should always be clear what has been added to what), the point is finally to destroy the definitive distinction between the two; prosthetics do not work unless they can efface themselves as such. The truly reassembled man was thus a consummate dissembler. A man with two artificial legs and a partially prosthetic hand reported, "I have met with strangers that never suspected any thing of me being artificial"; and one wearing limbs for amputations above the knee and elbow proclaimed, "Although my walk is slightly defective, many persons whom I frequently meet have no idea of my being so *largely* artificial" (Marks, *Patent* 207, 195). In the superficial logic of prosthetics, what matters is not who—or what—you are on the inside, but the impression you make on others. As manufacturers were quick to argue, the amputee owed it to himself (and to them) to keep up appearances—at around one hundred dollars apiece, state-of-the-art limbs cost about twice as much as clunkier makes.[33]

Among all the innovations in prosthetic technology during the nineteenth century, A. A. Marks's patent rubber foot stands out as the supreme simulation of human flesh.[34] Silencing the telltale stumping and squeaking of wooden legs and adding a spring to the step that mimicked the natural gait, the rubber foot produced an uncanny imitation of real ones. "My gait is so nearly natural," one customer wrote, "that many will not believe without actual inspection that art has in my case pieced out nature. My occupation makes me a traveling man, and I assure you I appreciate the rubber feet, whose easy, springy motion takes away half the terrors that come from the loss of limbs" (Marks, *Patent* 195). Hinging on a tension between assembly and authenticity—Rowley's catalogue referred to the wearer as the "Man Re-built," and one company even manufactured "Essential Limbs"—the artificial limb was promoted as a "substitute for nature" (Rideing 783); it was supposed, paradoxically, to be able to make the amputated body as good as new.[35] "I can do any thing with this leg. After ten days it became natural to me," wrote one satisfied customer, while another reported that "it is so long since I had my naturals that I have entirely forgotten them, and feel about as well off with the Marks' substitutes as I would had I those which nature gave me" (Marks, *Patent* 213, 193). Prosthetics could actually stand in for missing pieces, filling in anatomical gaps by fleshing out the illusion of flesh itself. At once absolutely material and totally make-believe—necessary but not essential—the artificial limb was practically too good to be true.

Confusing the relationship between essence and imitation (ironically by imitating too well), artificial limbs ultimately instantiated a problem of ontological priority—in duplicating flesh they ended up displacing it. As one wearer wrote of his rubber feet, "the only trouble with them is that they are too near like my natural feet for my own good" (Marks, *Patent* 195). Equating rubber with flesh and wood with bone (as if to suggest that for all practical purposes they were essentially the same), Rowley argued that "the natural foot and the Rowley foot are built alike, as each has a solid internal foundation. Each have the outer elastic covering to give it form and to serve as a cushion on which to tread." "Elastic, resilient, noiseless and natural in appearance" (Rowley 18), rubber could mimic the "elasticity" of human flesh because flesh already resembled rubber. Rubber even seemed in some ways to improve on flesh. Limb makers were quick to point out that as lifelike as they were in other ways, rubber feet never smelled (they were "as odorless as wood" and were "sealed up in a solid covering which would prevent the emanation of an odor, if one did exist" [Rowley 22]). They also never aged ("We have old rubber feet, made from sponge stock like we now use, which have been used from twelve to fifteen years, and they are not hard nor have they lost their elasticity" [Rowley 22]). Wooden legs, by contrast, made poor substitutes because they were anatomically incorrect—their "bony foundation is all on the outside" (Rowley 18). Once essence is defined as capability, and once what matters—in all senses of the word—is understood to be what is useful, or, more specifically, as what is actually being used, it ceases to be clear just what or where the prosthetic is, and how or whether it differs from the flesh it is replacing.

At once lifelike and larger than life—the rubber foot was "the king of all other feet" (Marks, *Patent* 200)—artificial limbs ultimately set the standard they were standing in for. Indeed, the very acknowledgment that prosthetics were "not of course equal [to] Nature's handiwork" (Rowley 174) encodes an understanding of the body as secondary to its own substitution by imagining essence as artifact, the material manifestation of a mechanical ideal (one newspaper even referred to human legs as "natural pedestals" [reprinted in Marks, *Patent* 153]). Conflating questions of autonomy and automation as a matter of routine, the language surrounding artificial limbs consistently confounds prosthetics with personality. As if they had lives, or even minds, of their own, artificial limbs often figure more as independent entities than as inanimate objects: one physician described his artificial limb's phenomenal performance in terms that granted it an agency unto itself—"Since it left your sales room my Rowley leg has walked an average of twenty miles per day, seventy-three hundred miles per year, or seventy-three thousand miles during the past ten years" (Rowley 163). A good artificial limb is self-motivated. It doesn't need a body to get it going—it "stands alone in a class by itself" (Rowley 38). Badly made limbs, by contrast, are totally unstable: "They seemed to be imbued with the spirit of the devil," one wearer proclaimed; "they always broke down at [the] most inopportune times" (Rowley 174). Good or bad, artificial limbs occasionally get carried away—a popular ballad called "The Cork Leg" tells the story of a man whose limb ran amok:

> He walk'd thro' squares and pass'd each shop,
> Of speed he went to the utmost top;
> Each step he took with a bound and a hop,
> And he found his leg he could not stop!

Refusing to halt when the wearer wanted to ("He clung to a lamp-post to stop his pace, / But the leg wouldn't stay, but kept on the chase"), the leg eventually wears its wearer out:

> He ran o'er hill and dale and plain,
> To ease his weary bones he'd fain;
> Did throw himself down but all in vain;
> The leg got up and was off again.

> He walk'd of days and nights a score;
> Of Europe he had made the tour:
> He died—but though he was no more,
> The leg walk'd on the same as before.
>   (Reprinted in Marks, *Patent* 171–72)[36]

Positioning the body itself as prosthesis (the amputee is, after all, only so much baggage dragging the cork leg down), the song suggests that mechanical parts cannot complete people without competing with them. Just as the limbs systematically supplant the subjects they are supposed to supplement, the discourse of prosthesis absolutely scrambles questions of ownership and identity (the problem with the maniacal leg, for instance, is precisely that it is possessed).

The parable of the cork leg finds a striking parallel in the athletic competitions held for wearers of artificial limbs, in which the question of just who—or what—was competing was entirely uncertain. Pitting amputees with comparable disabilities against one another, these contests functioned primarily as economic competitions among commodified bodies; they measured manliness in feet and inches (the record for the standing broad jump was six feet four inches, set at the annual meeting of the National Association of Railway Surgeons in 1895 [Rowley 110]), and they awarded prizes to both the athlete and the manufacturer of his limbs—as if to say that each played an equal part in the victory. Ultimately defining the amputee's worth in terms of his ability to beat out other brands of men, the ethos of these tournaments was implicitly "may the best make win." George B. Iliff, for instance, ran away with the all-around title at the 1897 meeting of the National Association of Railway Cripples; wearing two of Rowley's artificial legs, Iliff won the one-hundred-yard dash, the running high jump, the mile walk, the mile bicycle race, the standing broad jump, and the half-mile bicycle race. He went on to become the "Man Re-built," the poster boy for Rowley's artificial legs (fig. 17).[37] Proving that dismemberment does not have to end in disability, and suggesting that as a consequence the loss of limbs need not result in a corresponding loss of self, these contests encapsulated the constructivist impulse of prosthetics. They not only promoted a model of self as an unassailable construct, but also pitted different constructions against one another in such a way as to disqualify those that were unable to compete (as one man wrote to Rowley, the Rowley leg "has all other artificial and some natural legs beaten to a 'frazzle'" [150]). In so doing, they staged—and celebrated—the notion that the natural body had become obsolete.

Positioning body and image as interchangeable parts, prosthetics ultimately fetishized flesh as fabrication: "We imagine that the wearers of

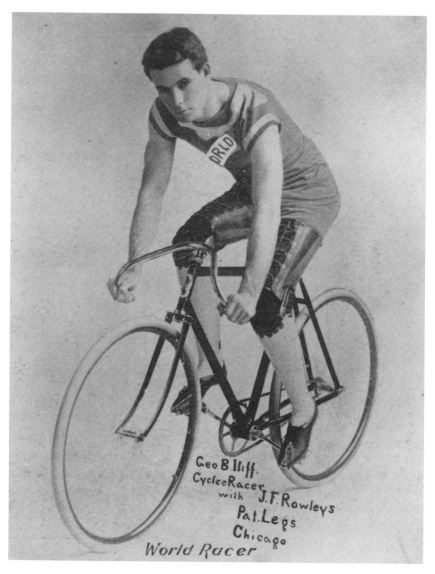

Fig. 17. George B. Iliff. From J. F. Rowley, *An Illustrated Treatise on Artificial Legs with Patent Wax Sockets* (1911).

these artificial limbs grow attached to them, as to a meerschaum pipe, and it occurs to us that there must be a large amount of satisfaction in taking one's leg off and rubbing it up and down in a fondling way" (Rideing 784). The division of the body into a series of "attachments" could be taken too far: "Some connoisseurs—for there are connoisseurs even in this—have collections of legs—week-day legs, Sunday legs, dancing legs, and riding legs, each expressly made for a distinct purpose. But this is vanity, and leadeth only unto vexation of spirit" (784). Nevertheless, the attraction of prosthetics was ultimately the concept of anatomy as apparatus. Prosthetics made the body optional, a known quantity that could be put on and taken off, incarnated and objectified at will.

> Coming home in the evening from a day of toil, and throwing himself into an arm-chair for a consoling smoke, [the wearer] can take off his boots and put on his slippers in the most natural manner possible. . . . [I]f he be of a utilitarian turn, with little care for trappings and seemings, he can discard the limb altogether when he is seated, and put it in a corner like an umbrella or a walking-stick. Or, if he has the native habit of sitting with his heels elevated above his body, he can continue to enjoy that delusive pleasure by resting his artificial leg on the window-sill while he sits upon the lounge in a more comfortable posture. A thousand advantages suggest themselves, and therein we find an example of the excellent law of compensation which atones for so many of our grievances. (Rideing 783)

The modern artificial limb could thus be both body and object, self and other at the same time. Delicately molded and covered with an enameled leather coating that passed for skin ("the form is perfection, the instep really arched, and the ankle trim. The calf swells with exquisite gradations, and recedes toward a well-shaped knee. The surface is smooth and glossy as satin, and delicately tinged"), it is designed to be a dead ringer for the real thing ("when we rap it with our knuckles it gives forth a hollow, sepulchral sound"). So it was that the discourse of prosthesis ultimately articulates a fantasy of dismemberment, a dream of not only being able to take the body off, but even of discarding the artificial limb itself as a kind of phantom, a signifier that doesn't signify: "The modern artificial leg is a complete illusion, and the wearer himself

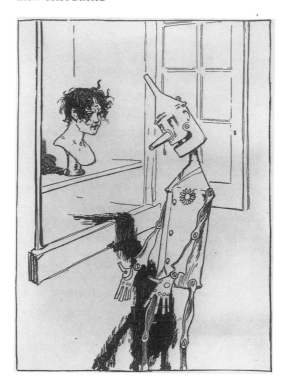

Fig. 18. The Tin Woodman meets his meat head. From L. Frank Baum, *The Tin Woodman of Oz* (1918).

may easily forget its unreality" (783–84). The obsession with putting the shattered body back together ends as a sort of detached fascination with the possibility of simply setting the whole thing aside (or at least in the corner with the umbrellas).

This fantasy of distantiation finds its most extreme incarnation in the figure of the Tin Woodman, L. Frank Baum's version of the Man Re-built.[38] Taking prosthetics past the breaking point by centering on a man made entirely of artificial parts (being wholly prosthetic, he cannot strictly be considered prosthetic at all), *The Tin Woodman of Oz* (1918) resolutely confuses the difference between original and imitation. Accidentally cutting himself to pieces with his own enchanted ax—legs first, then arms, followed by body, and finally by head—Nick Chopper is gradually made over from a "meat" body to a metal one by a local tinsmith who fashions artificial parts in exchange for the ones they are replacing. Asserting that identity cannot be dislocated as long as some body is in place—"A man with a wooden leg or a tin leg is still the same man; and, as I lost parts of my meat body by degrees, I always remained the same person as in the beginning, even though I was all tin and no meat" (29–30)—the story sees the body as profoundly inessential, simply a collection of disposable parts.[39]

Imagining what would happen if body and prosthesis could meet each other on their own terms, Baum stages a confrontation between the Tin Woodman and his ex-head, which he discovers on a stand in the tinsmith's cupboard: "'Good gracious!' cried the Tin Woodman in astonishment. 'If you are Nick Chopper's Head, then you are *Me*—or I'm *You*—or—or—What relation *are* we, anyhow?'" (212). The Head tries to pass him off as a poor relation, an inferior sort who is simply clamoring for recognition—"I'm not anxious to claim relationship with any common, manufactured article, like you. You may be all right in your class, but your class isn't my class. You're tin" (212). But the Woodman insists on a closer connection, defining the Head as his own, even though the two are no longer the same:

> "You belong to me," the Tin Woodman declared.
> "I do not!"
> "You and I are one."
> "We've been parted," asserted the Head. "It would be unnatural for me to have any interest in a man made of tin. Please close the door and leave me alone."
> "I did not think that my old Head could be so disagreeable," said the [Tin Woodman]. "I—I'm quite ashamed of myself; meaning *you*." (215)

The exchange exposes the basic paradox at the heart (if it only had a heart) of the logic of prosthesis: defining the essential body as the usable one, it puts flesh on a pedestal at the same time that it puts it away (fig. 18).

METAPHORS

So compelling was the artificial limb as a figure for liberation-through-technology that by the early decades of the twentieth century it had become a metaphor for technology itself. Writing in 1930, Freud himself turned the artificial limb into an elaborate rhetorical device, using it to describe the paradoxical process by which modern technologies both amplified the body and, in so doing, rendered that body increasingly obsolete:

> With every tool man is perfecting his own organs, whether motor or sensory, or is removing the limits to their functioning. Motor power places gigantic forces at his disposal, which, like his muscles, he can employ in any direction; thanks to ships and aircraft neither water nor air can hinder his movements; by means of spectacles he corrects defects in the lens of his own eye; by means of the telescope he sees into the far distance; and by means of the microscope he overcomes the limits of visibility set by the structure of his retina. In the photographic camera he has created an instrument which retains the fleeting visual impressions, just as a gramophone disc retains the equally fleeting auditory ones; both are at bottom materializations of the power he possesses of recollection, his memory. With the help of the telephone he can hear at distances which would be respected as unattainable even in a fairy tale. . . . Man has, as it were, become a kind of prosthetic God. When he puts on all his auxiliary organs he is truly magnificent; but those organs have not grown on him and they still give him much trouble at times. (41–43)[40]

Freud's happy comparison points to an actual historical correlation: modern artificial limbs were developed alongside the cameras, telephones, typewriters, X-ray machines, and primitive projectors of the late Victorian period. Prosthetics were both the material product of this historical moment and, as we have seen, a powerful figure for the moment itself. So powerful is that figure that we continue to use it today. In *Bodies and Machines* (1992), for example, Mark Seltzer takes prosthesis as a template for what he terms the late-nineteenth-century "body-machine complex," arguing that "the double logic" of technology "as prosthesis" expressed the "double logic of sheer culturalism," the simultaneously "panicked" and "exhilarated" proposition that "the individual is something that can be made" (157, 160). In so doing, Seltzer recapitulates the very Victorian logic he is discussing, abstracting the artificial limb into a metonymy for the identic tensions that characterized the era when artificial limbs themselves were being both modernized and metaphorized. The latter half of the nineteenth century thus not only marked the birth of technological modernity, but also laid the groundwork for what has become one of the defining conceptual formations of that modernity: the notion of "prosthesis" as both a metaphor for and materialization of a perfectly realized—if occasionally unwieldy—mode of (self) production.

As the example of Seltzer suggests, contemporary theorists routinely depend on prosthetic metaphors to articulate fantasies of agency. In *The Body in Pain* (1985), for instance, Elaine Scarry identifies prosthetics as a point of profound, even poetic, intersection between bodies and things: they cannot possibly "compromise or 'de-humanize' a creature who has always located his or her humanity in self-artifice" (253–54). Arguing that "the remaking of the human body is the ultimate aim of artifice," Scarry reads material culture as a romance based on a deep reciprocity between bodies and objects. Seeing artificial limbs and chairs as contributing equally to "the socialization of sentience," she asserts that every made thing may be seen as an expression of man's desire to amplify his own body, as a prosthetic extension of the self: "in making the world, man remakes himself" (255, 251). Most recently, "prosthesis" has become a favorite figure of that rapidly expanding subdivision of cultural studies, cybertheory. Cybertheory simultaneously makes the prosthesis into a trope for the hybridity of the modern world—"The postmodern state is clearly a prosthetic creature cobbled together out of various organic and cybernetic substances such as bioregions, cultures, markets, myths, histories, communities, and so on" (Gray and Mentor 244–45)—and uses it as a model for how to find pleasure and meaning within that world. To take just one example: *The Cyborg Handbook* (1995), edited by Chris Hables Gray, contains an essay by Sandy Stone entitled "Split Subjects, Not Atoms; or, How I Fell in Love with My Prosthesis," which romances a host of modern technologies—radios, transmitters, computers, motorcycles, plastic surgeries, telephones, but not, significantly, artificial limbs—as signs and sites of the peculiarly distantiated joys of our "prosthetic sociality" (397). Removed from the scene of amputation and lifted into metaphor, prosthetics have become postmodern philosophy. Indeed, in the anthology *Prosthetic Territories: Politics and Hypertechnologies* (1995), edited by Gabriel Brahm Jr. and Mark Driscoll, prosthesis takes shape as a celebratory catchword for the liberatory politics of cultural studies itself: "New movements (against racism, male-dominant capitalism, ideologies of progress, individualism, and the appropriation of labor and the earth as mere 'resource,' or raw material) tend not to pause in dispute over the (im)purity of these regions. Nor do they agonize much over outdated divisions between 'theory' and 'practice.' Rather, they begin by assuming hybridity in all things. In an attempt to provisionally name this new terrain of political and cultural struggle, we have dubbed these hybrid spaces of theory-practice 'prosthetic territories' " (1).[41] Together, these examples point to an unsettling convergence between Victorian and contemporary thinking. In both nineteenth-century writing and recent efforts to theorize agency, "prosthesis" stands for a technology of selfhood that substantiates itself in and through technology. Although the politics of the postmodern critic are ostensibly fundamentally opposed to those encoded in nineteenth-century accounts of prosthetics, the two nevertheless appropriate the concept in markedly similar ways, deploying it as a model for a more or less idyllic materialism.

Following Freud (in this as in so many things), we have detached "prosthesis" from its origins in nineteenth-century thought, using it, paradoxically, to denote a release from the very conceptual structures it originally helped to materialize. For the Victorians, the prosthetic elision of man and machine was a means of conserving the status quo under the guise of physical, spiritual, and social liberation. Amputating prosthetics from their complex history as a Victorian technology of self in order to affix them metaphorically—prosthetically—to our own increasingly tenuous fictions of self-determination, we have managed not to notice that prosthetics originally enabled the logic they now appear to transcend. So it is that a central rhetorical apparatus of cultural studies—the metaphorical machinery it uses to advance some of its most adventurous theoretical transgressions—appears not to be so very far removed from Victorian invocations of prosthetics as a utilitarian mode of being. Indeed, we might even read our own dematerialization of prosthetics as the fullest realization of the liberal logic originally set in motion by Victorian artificial limbs.[42] In order to salvage shattered ideals of manliness, Victorians developed prosthetics that could build fractions of men into capable composite entities we would now identify as cyborgs. Today cyborgs are defined by their "prosthetic" relations to the material world. Like George Dedlow's oddly substantial phantom limbs, theory's prosthetics are phantasmatic projections, the metaphoric extensions of a materialist rhetoric that wants to uncover a stable way to ground that spectral character, the self, in a world where the concept of identity can no longer stand unproblematically on its own.

❦ FOUR
Monsters, Materials, Methods

In 1848, the British weekly *Punch* published a note on "Deformito-mania," a new social disease characterized by an almost insatiable fascination with freaks (fig. 19). "The walls of the Egyptian Hall in Piccadilly are placarded from top to bottom with bills announcing the exhibition of some frightful object within, and the building itself will soon be known as the Hall of Ugliness," the note laments. "We cannot understand the cause of the now prevailing taste for deformity, which seems to grow by what it feeds upon. . . . We understand that an exhibition consisting of the most frightful objects in nature is about to be formed at the Egyptian Hall, under the . . . title of the Hideorama. Poor Madame Tussaud, with her Chamber of Horrors, is quite thrown into the shade by the number of real enormities and deformities that are now to be seen, as the showmen say, 'Alive! alive!' Her wax is snuffed out, or extinguished, by the new lights now shining in Piccadilly, where a sort of Reign of Terror just now prevails" (90). As the term *deformito-mania* suggests, Victorians were mad about monstrosity: freaks of every description were a source of tremendous public interest throughout the century, drawing crowds at exhibition halls, museums, and circuses and providing the featured entertainment at exclusive social gatherings. Deformity was big business during the nineteenth century: P. T. Barnum made his fortune exhibiting "living curiosities" at his

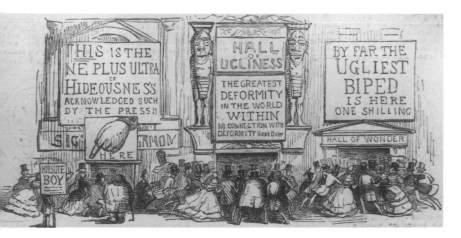

Fig. 19. "The Deformito-mania." From *Punch* (1848).

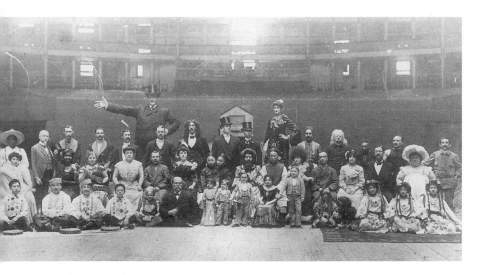

Fig. 20. Barnum and Bailey circus sideshow. Courtesy of the Circus World Museum, Baraboo, Wisc.

American Museum, while charismatic freaks such as Tom Thumb and the Siamese Twins became celebrities in their own right. So thoroughgoing was the mania for deformity that just about any physical anomaly was a viable commodity: excessive girth, unusual height, albinism, skinniness, and hairiness could all be the means of making a modest living (fig. 20). Freaks were in high demand, wanted dead or alive: if a peep at a live freak could cost as little as a few pence, a dead one could be worth hundreds of pounds. Medical men contracted with showmen and undertakers for the corpses of freaks, dissected them, and placed their articulated skeletons on display in pathological museums.[1] The source of almost bottomless curiosity, deformity provided a sensory distraction, a resource of delight and disgust that never ceased to be exciting and new. As infinitely varied as nature itself, deformity was never boring; it never dulled the senses; rather, the initial shock of looking could be endlessly recaptured and renewed. Deformito-mania speaks to a structure of imaginative dependency, a self-consciously irrepressible need on the part of an entire culture to contemplate deformity in all its phases: to stare at twisted, contorted, and aberrant bodies; to jeer at them; to speak to them; and even to touch them—again and again.

This chapter analyzes the symbolic importance of deformity for Victorian culture, showing how the spectacle of disfigurement ministered to a historically specific need to interrogate the contours of human identity.[2] Although "monsters" had occupied a privileged place in the Western imagination for hundreds of years, interest in them peaked during the nineteenth century, when industrialism and imperial expansion placed new pressures on traditional models of selfhood. The Victorian take on freaks differed qualitatively from the time-honored custom of showing human monsters at fairs alongside learned pigs and five-legged cows and adopting the occasional charismatic dwarf as a court pet. First, the shape and scope of the sideshow changed dramatically in response to opportunities presented by an emergent mass market. Like so many other marginal occupations, monstrosity was professionalized during the nineteenth century and became the first truly international entertainment industry. All the world was a potential audience, and showmen such as P. T. Barnum capitalized on the increasing ease of travel and advertising to great effect: with their world tours and widespread fame, figures such as Tom Thumb became some of the earliest superstars. Second, the symbolic content of the show came to reflect the imaginative needs of a culture in a violent, chronic state of flux. Monsters were a liminal space, a place where increasingly problematic distinctions between nature and culture, subject and object, and body and machine could become the raw material of a new, improved technology of being. Deformito-mania registers the conceptual shift in the way deformity was apprehended by English culture. As a name for a distinctly new form of madness (however facetiously invoked), it bespeaks the sheer modernity of the Victorian fascination with freaks, associating it with, and even seeing it as symptomatic of, the drastic changes that took place as England converted itself from a primarily rural, agrarian society into a mass culture of cities and machines.

It is no coincidence that the 1840s saw the advent of deformito-mania in England: this was also the decade in which England radically restructured itself in order to facilitate its emerging mass market, laying thousands of miles of railroad tracks, opening more and more factories, and repealing the Corn Laws in order to expand trade. Ambivalence was the operative word for the Forties: as commodities began flooding the markets like never before, Chartist agitation peaked, cholera killed thousands of people, thousands of starving Irish immigrated to England, and fears that "progress" was somehow profoundly inhumane began to shape social critique. Where cholera condensed a nightmare of dissolution into its symptoms, monsters managed the intense confusion generated by these dramatic shifts by compressing the massive political and social upheavals of the decade into the manageable and comic space of the show.

Etymologically, *monster* means "show" (also "warning" or "portent").[3] The monster was a show in an era of shows; its cultural work took shape not in the clinical logic of the case study, but rather in the lurid framework of public display.[4] Appearing amid an endless succession of panoramas, dioramas, light shows, peep shows, art exhibitions, fairs, and scientific demonstrations, freak shows imaged the paradox of personality in the age of consumer capitalism—not by displaying things, as museums, industrial exhibitions, and world's fairs did, but by displaying human beings *as* things, or "curiosities." Monsters were thoroughly commodified; they were selves whose idiosyncrasies were for sale, individuals whose defining features could be consumed by the hungry eyes of a public willing to pay for peeps. But even as commodities, monsters incorporated a fantasy of individuality. Deformity stood out in a world increasingly oriented around mechanization and routine. Every freak was unique, irreducible, intractable; freakish flesh was marvelously impractical, totally outside the automated logic of efficiency that molded the bodies of "normals" into standardized patterns of behavior. Owning themselves by selling themselves, freaks straddled the boundary between body and commodity by marketing their own misshapenness. In so doing, they called into question the status of any body—normal or not—in a world where everything could be bought and sold. In this respect, deformity constitutes a symbolic counterpart to the discourses of cholera, breast cancer, and dismemberment described in the previous chapters. Moving from case studies of particular pathologies to a more general analysis of bodily anomaly, this chapter shows how that comparatively broad category—monstrosity—provided a means of reinventing culture whose power lay, ironically, in its utter impracticability. Embodying a sort of twisted allegory for the birth of industrial modernity, deformity worked philosophically. Victorian monsters were physical analogies for the awful fascination of change, and as such their very defects served to pressure the concept of personhood into new, awkwardly optimistic shapes.

MONSTROUS OPTICS

Despite their popularity—or, more precisely, because of it—freak shows were at the center of a heated debate about the character of British culture. People worried that the rise of the freak show signified a decline in national judgment; they expressed concern that the "taste for the Monstrous" came at the expense of England's aesthetic sensibilities: "If *Beauty and the Beast* should be brought into competition in London, at the present day, *Beauty* would stand no chance against the *Beast* in the race for popularity. . . . There seems to be a sort of fascination in the horrible; and we can only hope, as the mania has now reached its extreme, a healthy admiration for the 'true and the beautiful' . . . will immediately begin to show itself" ("The Deformito-mania" 90). Deformito-mania thus described a maddening of taste. Victorian periodicals loudly lamented the traffic in "human excrescence and abortion," bewailing the fact that "beauty is no recommendation" to modern showmen, who "look out systematically for deformity, and earn their degraded beer through the medium of the mishaps of nature" ("Revelations of a Showman" 190). Critics argued that monsters had absolutely nothing to offer the cultivated gaze: "What advantage, what pleasure, what information can any one gather from an interview with a blinking Albino, whose eyes are as red as those of a ferret, and whose hair, ostentatiously combed over her shoulders, is as white as . . . snow? What charm can the most ardent votary of Bacon find in the conversation of the Pig-faced Lady? What coalitionist could brave the disgust engendered by a survey of the Pie-bald Girl?" ("Revelations of a Showman" 190). Assuming that the purpose of public exhibition ought to be to edify and improve, to entertain through instruction, journalism berated the sheer inutility of the freak show, its total want of intellectual and aesthetic content. With nothing to offer the trained eye, freaks were a gross insult to established standards of decorum, a monstrous offense whose magnitude was directly proportional to the degree of deformity displayed. Fat ladies, for example, far exceeded the limits of feminine beauty: "We do not object to a certain degree of *en-bon-point* in females; but, when they surpass the weight of twenty stone in the scales, they are anything but pleasant to look on." Likewise, giants were a vast assault on the senses. "A knock-kneed, ill-made, ungainly, unshapely, and preposterously stupid section of mortals," they were ugly beyond measure: "Look at one of them, and what do you see to admire? Has he the form of an Apollo, the front of a Jove, or even the brawn of a Hercules? Nothing of the sort. He is shaped like the monster in Frankenstein—his forehead is villainously low—and the calves of his legs, from long confinement, are as flaccid as the bladder in the interior of a well-kicked football" ("Revelations of a Showman" 190–91). The unsightly outgrowth of a gradual democratization of taste, the freak show was in every way a sign of poor public judgment. At a penny or two per peep, monsters were simply not worth looking at.

Victorian debates about the moral and aesthetic status of popular shows, particularly freak shows, grew out of a discussion that was hundreds of years old. What was new in the nineteenth century was how these long-standing concerns about cultural value got caught up with new anxieties about the specific impact of mass culture on the humanity of the English people. Commentators, appalled that an enlightened age could see disease as good theater, argued—largely unsuccessfully—that human pathology was a private tragedy, not a public performance. "Do you know that partial or faulty development is nothing but disease?"

one writer exhorted. "Let retirement be the lot of the being whom nature has prevented from mingling freely with its fellow-creatures. Let the brand be covered, the stigma hid. Let the secresy of private dwelling or public asylum enwrap it. Let us have no unfortunates—the victims at once of nature's mysterious displeasure—and the world's insolent and heedless curiosity" ("On the Disadvantages of Not Being a Dwarf" 329–30). Failure to distinguish between the beautiful and the ugly—between a show worthy of recognition and an eyesore—marked a kind of aesthetic aphasia on the part of the public, an utter incapacity to appreciate the need for such distinctions in the first place. Monsters helped produce a kind of collective apathy; the cheap thrill of bodily degeneration bespoke a vulgarity so profound, a public sensibility so dull, that it could not even register disease as disease. There was no sense of suffering associated with the show; the spectacle of deformity was apprehended as pure entertainment.

This pattern is perhaps best exemplified in the figure of Tom Thumb, P. T. Barnum's fabulously successful miniature man. In the spring of 1846, toward the end of a hugely lucrative two-year tour of Europe, Tom Thumb appeared at the Egyptian Hall in Piccadilly opposite Robert Haydon, a well-known English painter. Haydon, who had built a career as a historical painter, often showed his canvases in the Egyptian Hall while human oddities and curious acts were performing in other rooms, and he expected to earn enough from this show to pay off his debts and perhaps even put some money away. Barnum's tiny protégé was too much for Haydon, however, stealing his audience and drawing a huge crowd of his own. "They rush by thousands to see Tom Thumb," wrote Haydon. "They push, they fight, they scream, they faint, they cry help and murder, and oh, and ah. They see my bills, my boards, my caravans, and don't read them. Their eyes are open, but their sense is shut. It is an insanity, a rabies, a madness, a furor, a dream. I would not have believed it of the English people" (quoted in Fitzsimons 144). Embittered by what he saw as an unconscionable lapse of national perspective, Haydon ran a notice in the *Times* sardonically announcing the "*Exquisite Feeling of the English People for High Art.—* GENERAL TOM THUMB last week received 12,000 people, who paid him £600; B. R. HAYDON, who has devoted 42 years to elevate their taste, was honored by the visits of 133½, producing £5 13 6" (the half

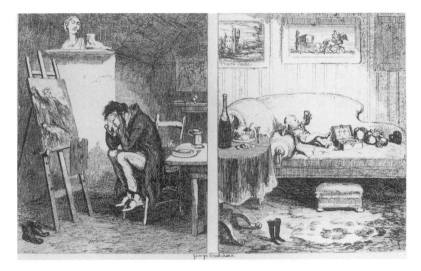

Fig. 21. "Born a Genius and Born a Dwarf," by George Cruikshank. From *Cosmic Almanack* (1847).

person, he noted, was a little girl) (quoted in Altick 414). Demoralized and deeply in debt, Haydon committed suicide a few weeks later. Haydon's death crystallized anxieties about the decline of the English character. The *Times* wrote that "the display of a disgusting dwarf attracted hordes of gaping idiots, who poured into the pockets of a Yankee showman a stream of wealth one tithe of which would have redeemed an honourable English artist from wretchedness and death. . . . These are the events which compel even sober-minded men towards the conviction that this condition of society should no longer exist, whatever be the cost of the change" (quoted in Fitzsimons 144–45) (fig. 21).[5]

Staging the displacement, and even destruction, of high English art by cheap American amusement, Tom Thumb materialized deep-seated anxieties about the capacity of English culture to survive the rise of the mass market. So thoroughly was the dwarf identified with the threat posed to English markets by foreign goods that *Punch* lampooned him as an argument against free trade: "In consequence of the success of General Tom Thumb, diminutiveness appears to have come into fashion, and we have not only an English Thumb, but a Spanish speculator has imported a Thumb for the purpose of having a dip into John Bull's pocket. . . . The fact is, there appears to be a regular glut of

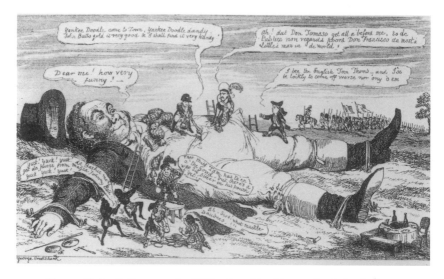

Fig. 22. "John Bull among the Lilliputians," by George Cruikshank. From *Comic Almanack* (1847).

Dwarfs, or Dwarves, at this particular time, and there is some danger of overstocking the market. We are surprised that an agitation is not commenced on behalf of native littleness, calling upon the Government to lay a heavy tax upon the foreign article" ("More Dwarfs" 93). An American dwarf who cornered the English market for deformity during a period of intense controversy over economic policy, Tom Thumb exemplified the dangers inherent in unregulated competition (1846 was not only the year that Tom Thumb drove Robert Haydon to suicide, it was also the year the Corn Laws were finally repealed). *Punch* even recommended that a protective tariff be placed on Tom Thumb, a tax that would clearly demarcate him as a "raw article of American produce" (93). George Cruikshank echoed *Punch*'s concerns in an 1847 etching depicting a bemused John Bull having his pockets emptied by a swarm of foreign dwarves while an unemployed English dwarf looks unhappily on (fig. 22).

As the example of Tom Thumb suggests, monsters enabled Victorians to articulate diffuse anxieties about the ability of English subjects to apprehend and evaluate their world intelligently. Social critics worried openly about the political consequences of vulgarity, arguing that the popularity of monsters laid bare an almost crippling lack of social vision. Thomas Carlyle, for instance, openly berated a society that would spend money to look at freaks of nature even as it refused to recognize—let alone repair—widespread social ills: "May we not well cry shame on an ungrateful world . . . which will waste its optic faculty on dried Crocodiles, and Siamese Twins?" (*Sartor Resartus* 205). Writing in 1831, at the height of Reform Bill fervor, Carlyle used the sensation caused by the Siamese Twins' 1829 tour of England to drive home his point about the questionable values of his culture. Suggesting that the freak show was a shameful distraction, a terrible waste of the English capacity to see, Carlyle posited a causal link between the observational powers of the public and the production of political energy. In his formulation, "optic faculty" and the capacity for purposeful action are conjoined (rather like the Siamese Twins themselves). The danger of indiscriminate looking is that certain hideous sights—mummified remains, monstrous births—can incapacitate the observer, absorbing his attention so totally that the reformist potential contained within his "optic faculty" is, along with the price of admission, carelessly thrown away.

For Carlyle and other critics, the problem with monsters was that they solicited a distinctly uncultivated, uncritical gaze. "Whet[ting] the public appetite for wonder" ("Barnum" 219), their mass appeal lay in their capacity not only to "attract the mob" ("The Gratuitous Exhibitions of London, No. II" 194), but to stop the mob in its tracks. People didn't think about what they saw in monsters; they were merely arrested by the monsters themselves. Spending upward of a shilling per visit to see giants and dwarves, bearded women and armless men, boys fat and thin, people flocked to shows. There they were left speechless, able only to squint and stare at the spectacle of deformity. The freak show was an overpowering sensory experience, a scene of sheer physical apprehension: curiosities overwhelmed curious crowds; wonders inspired wonder; marvels were marveled at. Basking in a profoundly inarticulate gaze—what *Punch* called a "gaping ignorance" ("The Gratuitous Exhibitions of London: Preliminary" 179)—monsters inspired an entirely incoherent astonishment. Indeed, according to one article, the "bonafide prodigy" is the one with "no conceivable mission to accomplish" except to take everyone's breath away. True monsters were pure shock value: they seemed to have been "expressly created to make the universe 'stare and gasp'" (Costello 499). Monstrosity comprised the complex relation between physical aberration and its apolitical effects: the spectacle of human defect could disable the spectator, mar his objective distance, leave him incapable of knowing what he saw. Exhibiting a remarkable tendency to defuse the productive energy of others, monsters filled their critics with the fear that deformity dumbed the public down, absorbing it in a useless contemplation, a specularity that spent itself on bodies that weren't worth the wonder they inspired.

Wonder was of enormous value in itself, however, a bodily necessity so hard to come by that it was becoming a rarity in its own right. Automation, discipline, routine: all these things crowded wonder out of daily life. In his *Emotions and the Will* (1859), the psychologist Alexander Bain theorizes wonder as a moment of necessary sensory arrest, an intensely physiological sensation that instantaneously startles the individual out of the fixed patterns of his mental existence: "There is pre-supposed a certain routine, or use and wont, which the mind is prepared to expect, and receives with calmness or composure. The rupture of this accustomed continuity of events causes a certain shock which we denominate surprise, wonder, or astonishment. The accompanying circumstances may be very various; the breach of expectation being sometimes agreeable, and at other times very much the reverse" (67). Whether enjoyable or not (and wonder was, most often, "without much delicacy, sweetness, or charm . . . rather a coarse pleasure, like mere intensity of sensation, or violent bodily exercise" [69]), wonder was a necessary antidote to the "automatism of habit" that characterized so much modern experience (Foucault, *Discipline and Punish* 135). In a materialist economy increasingly dedicated to explaining away the inexplicable, the spectacle of deformity enabled an almost ritualistic renewal of an increasingly elusive emotion. Wowing the public again and again, the freak show provided a distinctly modern experience of awe, a cheap thrill that could be supplied on demand. The freak show was a utilitarian source of amazement, a standard procedure for lifting people out of their everyday ruts.

Moreover, the wonder inspired by monsters was not without content: the empty stares of awed observers were not devoid of meaning. A rapt gaze is inevitably a receptive one—it may not like what it sees, but it is compelled to keep looking all the same. I want to argue that those vacant gazes were useful symbolic spaces, that far from being a waste of "optic faculty," midgets, giants, dwarves, bearded women, fat men, albinos, fire-eaters, contortionists, living skeletons, and conjoined twins performed an important office in the formation and refinement of modern sensibilities. The tremendous pull of the monstrous physique suggests that it was in fact deeply meaningful, that far from being a useless, debilitating diversion, the spectacle of human disfigurement was doing substantial cultural work. The freak's ability to draw crowds where high art could not indicates not that monsters were consuming people's capacities for aesthetic appreciation and political action, as some Victorian critics would have it, but, more profoundly, that the spectacle of disfigurement spoke to people in ways traditional forms of art could not. Indeed, the spectacular utility of the freak show lay in its mute vulgarity. Monsters staged the unspeakable in the inarticulate space of communal wonderment, shaping the modern subject as a ridiculous figure, an absurd caricature of itself.

What made monsters so useful was precisely that they were reductive—fascinatingly, disgustingly, charmingly able to oversimplify the world. Tom Thumb, for instance, was imaged as a kitschy condensation of all mankind, a "chemical synthesis, in which manhood had been boiled down" (quoted in Kunhardt 51). A genuine imitation of masculinity at large, Tom Thumb belittled great traditions by compressing them into the fantastic littleness of his own body (fig. 23). Striking classical poses and impersonating such heroic figures as Napoleon and Frederick the Great, he made a mockery of the very concept of the noble pursuit: when asked by Wellington why he played such a pensive Napoleon, he replied, "I was thinking of the loss of the Battle of Waterloo" (quoted in Saxon 130). "A man in miniature," a "*mite* of humanity" (Barnum 257), his power lay precisely in his shrill, stilted speech and jerky little movements. "Like a wax-doll gifted with the power of locomotion" (Barnum 257), Barnum's dwarf was an image of manufactured humanity, an automaton, a toy. As a "commodity" that Barnum had "made to order," Tom Thumb's individuality was inseparable from his mechanical affect (quoted in Harris 309). As such, he was instrumental in dramatizing a peculiar new cult of personality, a charisma that established itself, paradoxically, through the perfect execution of planned, canned behavior (fig. 24). In Tom Thumb we see absurdity as

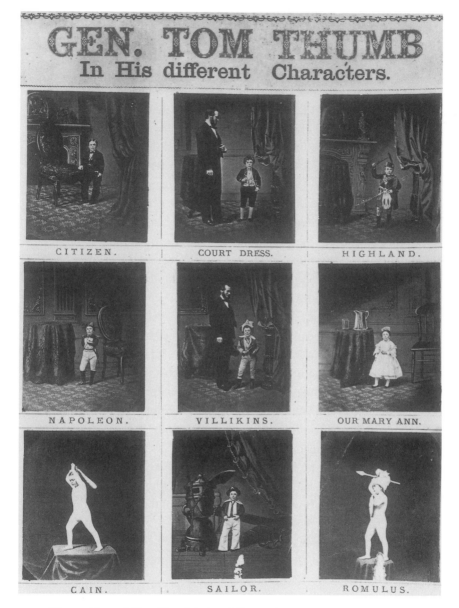

Fig. 23. General Tom Thumb in his different characters. Courtesy of the Barnum Museum, Bridgeport, Conn.

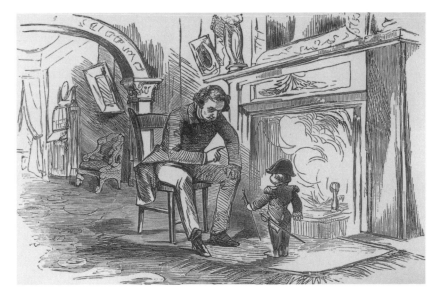

Fig. 24. Barnum training Tom Thumb. From P. T. Barnum, *The Life of P. T. Barnum*
(1855).

social strategy. He made millions for himself and Barnum as a self
without history, depth, or substance; a self that was instead constituted
as a slick surface of repetitive response (he was at his slickest when
playing up his penchant for kissing the ladies: a bargain at twenty-five
cents a pop). What Barnum was selling was not simply the sight of a
precocious American boy (indeed, he exhibited his charge as an English boy in America), but the oddly evacuated model of personhood
that this boy promoted, the riveting spectacle of manliness made ro-
botic, of the grand hero as a compact, portable machine.

In the freak show, the structure of distorted surprise metamor-
phosed into a hermeneutic of culture. Monsters gave shape to ideas in
ways that were beyond established modes of verbal and visual communication; at once incredible and actual, unbelievable and undeniably
real, they became metaphors for the impossible character of modern
life. Over the course of the nineteenth century the grossly deformed
came to image the convolutions of progress, their variously stunted and
skewed physiques providing an apt figure for the irregular and unpredictable process of change itself. With their missing limbs and extra
parts, spotted skin and misshapen flesh, monsters displayed a remark-

able capacity for defamiliarizing the status quo. So thoroughgoing was the sense of the freak as a lens through which the world could be viewed that deformity itself became a metaphor for social perspective. William Thackeray, for instance, used giants and dwarves as figures for problems of analytical distance. In order to see the same old things from new angles, he wrote, "we have but to change the point of view, and the greatest action looks mean; as we turn the perspective-glass, and a giant appears a pigmy" (*History of Henry Esmond* 235). Monstrous optics did have their limits, however; as one physics book put it, "If a dwarf on the shoulders of a giant can see farther than the giant, he is no less a dwarf in comparison with the giant" (Grove 3).

By providing a new way of seeing, monsters ministered to a historically specific need to revise the contours of human identity.[6] On the broadest level, freaks provided an alternative viewpoint on basic questions about what it meant to inhabit a body, and, more broadly, on what it meant to be human. To return to the Siamese Twins Carlyle found so distracting—far from providing a specular experience that was devoid of symbolic content, conjoined twins occupied an important position in Victorian debates about personhood. People born bound together focused pervasive uncertainties about the mind's relation to the body, providing a curious but compelling angle from which to examine the nature of human autonomy, on the one hand, and the structure of formal relationships, on the other. Medical and popular fascination with conjoined twins centered on whether such entities were one person or two (figs. 25, 26). Joined twins had unique personalities that were capable of fighting with each other (Chang and Eng occasionally came to blows) and even of falling in love (the Siamese Twins married sisters and fathered twenty-two children). With different tastes (Chang drank, Eng abstained), different talents (Chang was sociable, Eng intellectual), and different tolerances (Eng couldn't hold Chang's liquor), they were two fully formed selves living in a body that wasn't big enough for both of them. The twins couldn't live with one another (they kept separate households), but they also couldn't live without each other (doctors didn't dare separate them surgically for fear of the consequences). Neither this nor that, not self but not other, their lives were an elaborate negotiation of personal boundaries; joined at the chest, they were stuck with each other; anatomically enmeshed (they

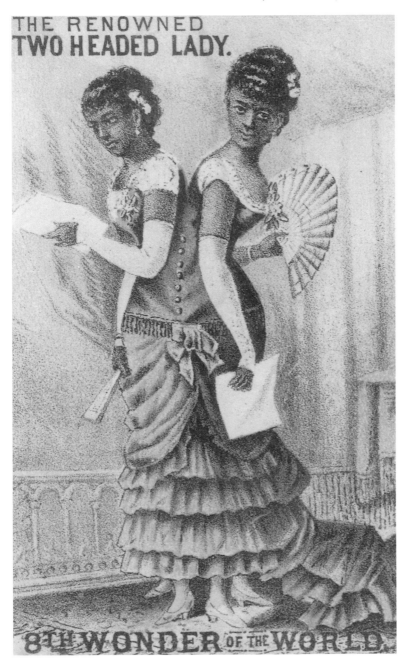

THE RENOWNED
TWO HEADED LADY.

8TH WONDER OF THE WORLD.

Fig. 25. Millie-Christine, the Renowned Two-Headed Lady. Courtesy of the College of Physicians, Philadelphia.

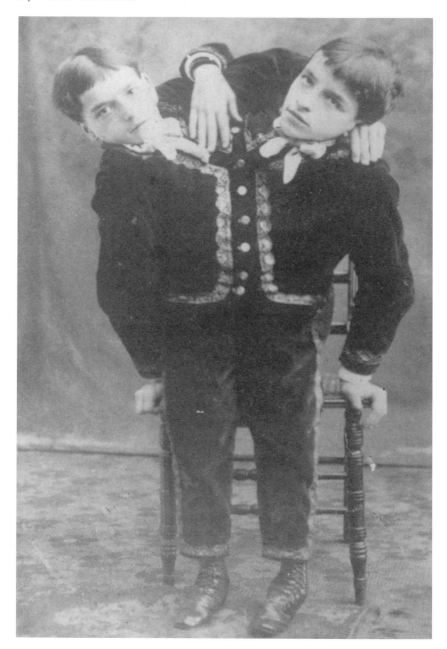

Fig. 26. The Tocci Brothers. Courtesy of the College of Physicians, Philadelphia.

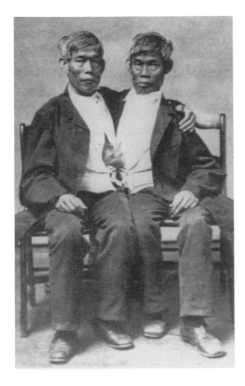

Fig. 27. Chang and Eng.
Courtesy of the Circus World
Museum, Baraboo, Wisc.

shared a double liver and lots of connective tissue), they were phys-
iological co-dependents living for, in, and through each other (when
Chang had a stroke, Eng had to support his paralytic body; when
Chang died in his sleep, Eng expired soon after) (fig. 27).[7]

Pulling apart the structure of personhood, the twins provided a
means of shaping social commentary. Their deformity operated as a
conceptual tool, an anatomically incorrect way of making analytical
connections. Specifically, the band of skin that bound the brothers
together became a metaphor for impossible, impractical unions. Mark
Twain made the twins into a satire on secession, using them to illustrate
the absurdity of cutting up the United States: "During the War [the
twins] were strong partisans, and both fought gallantly all through the
great struggle—Eng on the Union side and Chang on the Confederate.
They took each other prisoners at Seven Oaks, but the proofs of capture
were so evenly balanced in favor of each, that a general army court had
to be assembled to determine which one was properly the captor and
which the captive. The jury was unable to agree for a long time; but the

vexed question was finally decided by agreeing to consider them both prisoners, and then exchanging them" ("Personal Habits of the Siamese Twins" 209). Where Twain made the Siamese Twins into a metaphor for a divided nation, a union defined by its difference from itself, feminist writer Frances Power Cobbe used them to support a scathing critique of English marriage laws. The notion that husband and wife are "one flesh," she reasoned, is preposterous and ought not to be invoked as an argument against divorce. Unlike the "Siamese twins, who are tied together—not by Mother Church but by Mother Nature—so effectually that [doctors] are . . . powerless to release them," married couples are not bound by anything except ridiculous laws. Moreover, these laws put women at a financial disadvantage compared to which the Siamese Twins are quite well off. Whereas married women are entirely dispossessed, the Siamese Twins enjoy a strictly egalitarian arrangement: "Each of them has . . . the satisfaction of dragging about his brother as much as he is dragged himself; and if either has a pocket, the other must needs have every facility of access thereto" (122). Cobbe was not alone in seeing the Twins' union as a commentary on marriage. The London *Examiner* wrote that twins suffered a fate worse than marriage: "The link which unites them is more durable than that of the marriage tie—no separation can take place, legal or illegal—no Act of Parliament can divorce them, nor can all the power of Doctors' Commons give them a release even from bed and board" (quoted in Grosz 63). Establishing a series of connections between deformity and society, the band of flesh that bound the brothers became the means of dissecting the social body; their famous "ensiform appendix" gained metaphoric dimensions over time, eventually coming to stand for some of the double binds that molded life in England and America.

Less a fatal distraction from relevant social issues than a strategic embodiment of the social, Victorian monsters materially conditioned critiques of culture. Monsters provided a means of thinking about the ontological distortions of modernity. They could be abstracted into rhetorical figures, enabling writers to anatomize bizarre cultural formations; and they were bizarre cultural formations in their own right, entrepreneurs who used the misfortune of their birth as the raw material of commercial venture, converting their defective bodies into viable commodities simply by making spectacles of themselves. This peculiar dynamic became the basis for a prominent thread in the extraordinarily varied vocabulary of Victorian deformity as monsters came increasingly to stand as figures for the vexed status of the human body under capitalism. Like the Siamese Twins, the Victorian freak was, conceptually speaking, a kind of two-headed monster, at once a product of the mass market (which could promote the deformed and pay them like never before) and an unspeakable allegory for how that market was distorting concepts of personhood almost beyond recognition. Monsters imaged the uncertain outline of an emergent commodity culture, their physical aberrations providing a frame of reference for the oddities—and possibilities—of progress.

MONSTROUS LOGICS

Wordsworth's description of Bartholomew Fair, quoted below, figures prominently in recent cultural criticism as an exemplary moment in nineteenth-century visual ideology.

> Above the press and danger of the crowd
> Upon some showman's platform
> . . . .
> All moveables of wonder, from all parts,
> Are here—Albinos, painted Indians, Dwarfs,
> The Horse of knowledge, and the learned Pig,
> The Stone-eater, and the man that swallows fire,
> Giants, Ventriloquists, the Invisible Girl,
> The Bust that speaks and moves its goggling eyes,
> The Wax-work, Clock-work, all the marvellous craft
> Of modern Merlins, Wild Beasts, Puppet-shows,
> All out-o'-the-way, far-fetched, perverted things,
> All freaks of nature, all Promethean thoughts
> Of man, his dullness, madness, and their feats
> All jumbled up together, to compose
> A Parliament of Monsters.
> (William Wordsworth, "The Prelude")

In *The Politics and Poetics of Transgression* (1986), Peter Stallybrass and Allon White look at this passage as a classic instance of bourgeois self-construction, a scene of looking that shapes a disciplined, disembodied middle-class subject from within the sanitizing space of analytic distance. For Stallybrass and White, the critical eye of the detached observer and the carnivalesque body of the low other are ideologically intertwined, entangled in a logic of othering in which the object of the gaze becomes, paradoxically, the source of the spectator's own inalienable selfhood. Tony Bennett showcases these same lines in *The Birth of the Museum: History, Theory, Politics* (1995), contending that in such passages one can trace the importance of the "exhibitionary complex" to the nineteenth-century disciplinary imagination. Bennett frames his argument as a refinement of Foucault's theory of panopticism, using the Victorian fetish for museums, shows, and fairs to contend that the act of looking was at least as important to the creation of the self-contained Victorian subject as the feeling that one was constantly being looked at. Both studies use Wordsworth's passage to illustrate logics of politicized sight, analyzing how nineteenth-century bourgeois subjectivity was consolidated through an optics of objectification. Each argues that Victorians learned about themselves by looking—in the one case by contemplating people, and in the other by viewing things. The one is a logic of othering, a strategy of seeing in which the subject is constituted by objectifying others; the other is a structure of educating, a demonstrative system of display in which the subject is constituted by critically examining instructive objects.[8]

In working to historicize the gaze that is currently so central to our thinking about power, Bennett and Stallybrass and White develop theories of bourgeois selfhood that assume a clear opposition between subjectivity and objectification: if the subject is formed by objectifying another, or by contemplating objects, objectification is, by implication, a means of depriving individuals of their status as subjects. This opposition has modulated much of the major recent work on nineteenth-century literature and culture, which tells the story of modern identity formation as the story of subjectivity: such varied work as Nancy Armstrong's *Desire and Domestic Fiction: A Political History of the Novel* (1987), Regina Gagnier's *Subjectivities: A History of Self-Representation in Britain, 1832–1920* (1991), John Kucich's *Repression in Victorian Fiction: Charlotte Brontë, George Eliot, and Charles Dickens* (1987), D. A. Miller's *The Novel and the Police* (1988), Mary Poovey's *Uneven De-*

velopments: The Ideological Work of Gender in Mid-Victorian England (1988), and Carolyn Steedman's *Strange Dislocations: Childhood and the Idea of Human Interiority, 1780–1930* (1995), to name a very few, all participate in the project of anatomizing the origins of the modern individual—a self broadly construed as a domesticated, psychologically complex subject. My observation that Victorian identity formation has been narrated as subject formation may seem tautological at first—but this is precisely my point. Our own association of selfhood with sub-jecthood is so firm that objectification operates for us as a synonym for the very worst kinds of oppression: to objectify, by today's definitions, *is* to dehumanize. I want to suggest that there is a species of anachronistic thinking at work here—that our own analytical models have so clouded our critical thinking that we have overlooked other ways the Victorians assembled selves. Monsters, for example, staged a model of self pro-foundly different from the one we are accustomed to hearing about, tracing a course of self-construction centered not on the gradual emer-gence of interiority, but rather on the production of exteriority, of self as a totally superficial entity, an eviscerated surface whose substance lies not in inner workings but in the contours of visibly distorted flesh. What was riveting about the freak show was the spectacle of self as object; it was the prospect of a selfhood compatible with—even im-manent in—those patterns of classification typically identified with the loss of self: commodification, mechanization, automation, routine. Part person, part imaginative device, the monster was a charismatic machine, a tool for imagining a type of individual whose humanity was not deadened by the monotonous rhythms of modern existence, but brought to life by them. Monsters make up a perverse subtext to master narratives of nineteenth-century identity formation, bringing to life a series of misbegotten figurations that had as their object the celebration of objectification itself.

Monsters were inextricably linked to things in the Victorian imagi-nation. The nineteenth-century freak show formulated a complex on-tology of identity formation in which the specular logic of othering is absolutely caught up in and refracted through contemporary fascina-tion with objects themselves. Displaying monsters alongside things, and frequently displaying them *as* things, the freak show framed an utterly literal form of objectification, a visual pattern in which the act of distantiated looking explicitly made the object of the gaze—a human being—into a metaphorical thing. In Wordsworth's description of Bartholomew Fair, for example, monstrous bodies and marvelous machines are arrayed alongside one another, as if to instance a basic structural affinity between the two. The parliament of monsters registers and arranges a formal taxonomy, a system of shapes whose figurative dimensions contrive a specular equivalency between the flawed body and the mechanical oddity. Misshapen flesh and "marvellous craft" have the same ocular, ontological status in the showman's display; indeed, as one in a series of "perverted things," misshapen flesh is, on some level, marvelous craft. For Wordsworth, then, the monster comprises not only the defective body, but also the coupling of that body with examples of modern invention.[9] The monstrosity here is the categorical transgression itself, the "parliament" formed by mating together distortion and contraption. It is the interpenetration of animate and inanimate forms, the equation of twisted physique and technical precision, the "jumbling up together" of gimmick and geek into a "far-fetched" composition, an ill-made still life of mismatched and yet strangely interchangeable parts.

We might take the hermeneutic structure of Bartholomew Fair as representative of nineteenth-century conceptions of monstrosity. As the century progressed, Wordsworth's specular logic, in which the monster stands as the sign of a conceptual miscegenation, a figure for the casual combination of subjects and objects, helped to focus diffuse anxieties about both the social status of things and the thingness of persons. As objects gained increasing social importance (as possessions), and as objectification emerged as a critique of industrialism (as a metaphor for a lost self-possession), the miscegenated materiality of the sideshow became a means of scrambling the distinctions between subject and object that were so vitally important elsewhere.[10] The sign of that scrambling, as we have seen, was the monster. At first glance, the use of the monster as an emblem for the hybridization of discrete forms—particularly those forms having to do with the differential classification of people and things—might seem to demarcate something like a critique of that hybridization. To say that mixing matter makes a monster is to suggest that the mixing itself is a monstrous gesture—an abortion, incapable of useful symbolic life. Such a reading is complicated, however, by the frankly happy, even gleeful, tone of the freak show. If the show made it possible to see the monstrous contiguity of people and things in consumer culture, it also openly celebrated the slippage between them. The freak show was above all else fun: able to turn a potential nightmare into a great time, monsters made a carnival of conceptual crisis, framing failures of imagination as festive, fabulous occasions.

P. T. Barnum's sideshows are the best example of this. More than any other showman, Barnum lifted the freak squarely into the nineteenth century.[11] When Barnum took over New York City's American Museum on January 1, 1842, the place was a moribund dusty repository of old bones, moth-eaten skins, moldering dioramas, and mediocre art. Within months Barnum had converted the museum into a hugely successful enterprise, tripling profits through skilled management, shameless promotion, and the peculiar blend of genuine instruction, unabashed humbug, and prurient appeal that was to become his trademark. Barnum intended the museum to be a comprehensive collection of the world's most unusual sights and interesting objects, a wonderfully diversified national gallery encompassing a "cyclopaediacal synopsis of everything worth seeing and knowing in this world's curious economy" (quoted in Fiedler 277). Part curiosity cabinet and part carnival, the American Museum fused the private collection and the itinerant show into a national monument, a cultural center that was a triumph of advertising and accumulation. Trading on an emergent mass public's insatiable desire to see and know the world (if only through the medium of exotic bits and pieces), Barnum took idiosyncrasy to unprecedented commercial heights. Effectively producing the curiosity as a corporate entity, the American Museum was big business; Barnum himself referred to it as "the largest and most complete 'Curiosity Shop' on [the North American] continent" (quoted in Saxon 16) (fig. 28).[12]

Barnum made millions displaying everything from articulated skeletons and stuffed birds to mummies, statues, and waxworks (among them a notoriously bad Queen Victoria). A dried mermaid and myriad Oriental artifacts were arrayed alongside scale models of famous scenes and landmarks; suits of armor and a collection of antique shoes shared space with a giant hairball taken from a sow's stomach, a piece of the

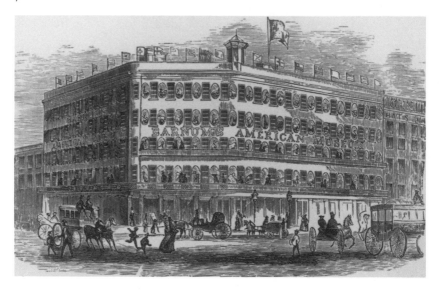

Fig. 28. Barnum's American Museum. From P. T. Barnum, *The Life of P. T. Barnum* (1855).

door of Columbus's birthplace, and a straw from the mattress the czar slept on at Buckingham Palace. The museum had a glassworks, a model steam engine, stuffed animals, and an in-house taxidermist who would prepare dead pets while the bereaved owners toured the premises. At different times the upper reaches of the museum housed a menagerie featuring lions, tigers, bears, ostriches, primates, and the first hippo seen in America; the lower floors held whales in enormous saltwater tanks (Saxon 92–94).[13] Barnum's greatest attraction, however, was his collection of human monsters, the marvelous troupe of giants, dwarves, fat ladies, thin men, albinos, bearded women, armless and legless wonders, and conjoined twins that he acquired, displayed, and, when necessary, replaced over the years. Billed as "living curiosities," Barnum's monsters were essentially mobile museum property. By day they stood alongside minerals, magnets, and optical instruments; at night they retired to the uppermost story of the vast museum, where they slept like so many precious possessions tucked safely away. Like the creaky mechanisms, deplorable artwork, and questionable artifacts cluttering the place, living curiosities occupied the status of wonderful junk. They were collector's items of dubious value, rarities of uncertain authenticity, fascinating stuff of inferior make. Treating human oddities as so many odds and ends, Barnum's curiosity shop framed deformity as a form of fabulous inutility; monsters were so much additional miscellany at the American Museum, poor things good for nothing but spectacular display.

Industrial exhibitions such as the one held at the Crystal Palace in 1851 were triumphs of organization: space was carefully subdivided by nation, product, and manufacturer. The result was a model material world, a global economy of made objects classified, qualified, and compartmentalized into an almost overwhelmingly orderly utopia. By contrast, Barnum's museum cultivated chaos. It was a scene of difference that refused to impose order on those differences, an artifactual explosion whose organizing principle was the utter absence of organization. A monument to diversity, Barnum's enterprise exhibited a weirdly multicultural materialism; it was a spectacularly democratic carnival that celebrated the uniqueness of anything and everything at once: "Industrious fleas, educated dogs, jugglers, automatons, ventriloquists, living statuary, tableaux, gipsies, albinoes, fat boys, giants, dwarfs, rope-dancers, caricatures of phrenology, and 'live Yankees,' pantomime, instrumental music, singing and dancing in great variety, (including Ethiopians) etc. Dioramas, panoramas, models of Dublin, Paris, Niagara, Jerusalem, etc., mechanical figures, fancy glass-blowing, knitting machines and other triumphs in the mechanical arts, dissolving views, American Indians, including their warlike and religious ceremonies enacted on the stage, etc., etc." (Barnum 225). Placing people, panoramas, bodies, beasts, ethnics, freaks, fancywork, and fabulous humbug side by side, Barnum installed a framework that essentially treated animals, vegetables, and minerals alike. Forging connections while leveling distinctions, Barnum's museum organized vastly different materials into an oddly homogeneous totality, a vision of culture whose seemingly infinite capacity for inclusion was matched—and mitigated—by its similarly awesome power to equalize the things it included. Difference was ultimately a system of *in*difference in Barnum's logic; monsters got lost in the shuffle as marvels became interchangeable, pieces in a series of substitutions whose seamlessness was arguably the most impressive wonder Barnum had to offer. The American Museum was an amazing mess, a semiotic system whose sloppy metonymies established equivalences among different wonders so as to deprive individual ones of an essential identity. By definition, a living curiosity is not a person—it is, rather, a qualitatively indistinct category. Part ugly body, part useless thing, the living curiosity is a doodad with a heartbeat, a whatchamacallit with attitude (at times, too much: Barnum threatened more than once to lock up his ornery albinos if they wouldn't behave themselves).

A monstrous analogy suggests itself here between Barnum's sidelong methods and the conceptual patterns of contemporary cultural studies, whose greatest gift and weakest link is precisely its capacity to argue by way of adjacency. Broadly speaking, cultural studies operates by putting seemingly disconnected things side by side and reading them through each other—Mark Seltzer describes this as a strategy of "drawing into relation," for example, while D. A. Miller invokes "conceptual cross-overs" and Lawrence Grossberg sees it as "articulation."[14] Whatever the specific vocabulary, this tactic is arguably constitutive of a branch of cultural studies that prides itself on its capacity to generate new readings of culture by way of a constructive, instructive clashing of seemingly disparate material. At the risk of simply mirroring the gesture I am wondering about, I want to suggest that this methodology participates in a politics of observation that is strikingly similar at times to the monstrous optics of the Victorian exhibition. Their analytical predicaments of the two are essentially analogous—what is often lost in the production of interesting cultural reflections, whether between objects or between objects of study, is precisely the capacity to articulate in historically convincing terms what those reflections might mean. In establishing a series of associations between malformed bodies and other cultural materials, deformity performed a kind of cultural theory, marking and manipulating some of the central epistemological problems of an emergent commodity culture. And like so much cultural theory, monsters dramatized ontological connections by allowing the material conditions of those connections to drop out of sight: what gets lost in the symbolic economy of Victorian monsters is, ironically, the materiality of the monster itself.

For Wordsworth, the monster is ultimately the sign of formal chaos. In his lines on Bartholomew Fair, monstrous bodies fade into the background as a conceptual monster, one that governs the sloppy whole of the fair's disorderly arrangements, comes to the fore. At Barnum's

American Museum, monsters stood less as the sign of an indiscriminate materialism's grotesque groupings than as their residual trace: what is striking about the museum is how thoroughly human deformity blended in there, how utterly it ceased to stand for and as itself. Etymologically, the word *freak* had extracorporeal dimensions before it had anatomical import: according to the *Oxford English Dictionary*, Milton coined the term as a synonym for *fleck;* his freak was a speck of color. And during the eighteenth century, freak as fleck became freak as flight of fancy, an odd impulse or whim. When the freak became a body in 1847, it necessarily contained the outlines of its earlier meanings. Layered onto the monster-freak was the sense of the freak as sign or marker—a brilliant spot; layered on as well was the sense of the freak as caprice, a sudden change of heart. Barnum's freaks scrambled all these senses together; striking signs of fickle times, they traced the deformed as oddly intractable traces, the remarkable unmarked markers of a subject position that was being progressively effaced, displaced, and replaced by a newly invented system of objects.[15]

In Wordsworth, monsters are leveled even as they stand for the effects of leveling; in Barnum's museum, the leveling is complete. No longer monsters, living curiosities were of a piece with the trumped-up treasures of the world's largest "curiosity shop," a "hall of wonders" whose most special effect was its capacity to establish such powerful specular and experiential equivalencies among its "diverse attractions" that visitors were as thrilled to leave as they were to arrive (eager crowds flocked to see the "egress," whose location was announced by a bright sign hung over the exit door). In Barnum's museum, and elsewhere in Victorian life, the monster virtually disappeared—like one of the dissolving views that were so popular throughout the century, monsters manifested themselves most strikingly in the act of fading away. Thin men, or living skeletons, stood out most clearly as disappearing acts. One such ethereal specimen was billed as the "Living Phantom," "whose body is so thin that it is almost transparent" (quoted in Saxon 101). Another showed himself as "the transparent man," shining electric light through his wasted members to demonstrate the sheer nature of his not-so-solid flesh (Gould and Pyle 603–4) (fig. 29).

Of course, it was not a literal disappearance. Indeed, the century's expansive fascination with fat attests to the monster's tremendous ca-

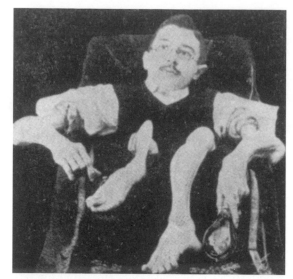

Fig. 29.
"Transparent Man."
From George M.
Gould and
Walter L. Pyle,
*Anomalies and Curi-
osities of Medicine*
(1901). Courtesy of
the College of
Physicians,
Philadelphia.

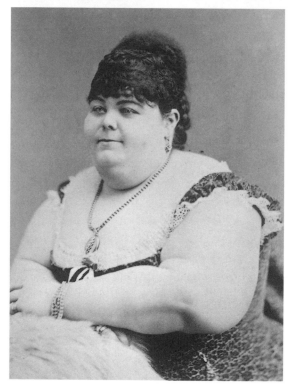

Fig. 30. Fat lady.
Courtesy of the
Becker Collection,
Syracuse University,
Syracuse, N.Y.

pacity to embody a totally inalienable presence (fig. 30). Monsters were nothing if not materially grounded. Nevertheless, the monster suffered a sort of symbolic erasure in shows such as Barnum's, which framed it as what could not be understood as itself.[16] The physical density of the monstrous body—its palpable uncertainty—was instead apprehended as a density of disparate associations. Take Daniel Lambert, for example, the most famous fat man of the nineteenth century. Weighing it at "above 50 stone, 14 pounds to the stone," and measuring "3 Yards 4 Inches round the Body, and 1 Yard One Inch round the leg, 5 feet 11 Inches high" (Altick 254), Lambert's size gave him great symbolic scope. In the early years of the century he made a tremendous John Bull, dwarfing the Napoleonic threat while embodying an England able to quash any challenge France might pose (figs. 31, 32). Later, he became both a symbol of urban sprawl ("London," George Meredith remarked, "was a Daniel Lambert of cities") and an image of massive mental power: Herbert Spencer once described a revered thinker as "a Daniel Lambert of learning." Famous during his own lifetime for his prodigious size and strength (at 739 pounds he was said to be an excellent swimmer and sportsman), Lambert's metaphorical feats outlasted his physical ones. Dead in 1809 of fatty degeneration of the heart, he lived on as a kind of thick description, an immensely layered trope for both the sizable convulsions of the modern world and the stabilizing power of weighty allusion. To figure Lambert as England is to make England immovable, invincible, to solidify its identity as a world power with massive metonymical force. To compare London to Lambert is to conjure solace by association; it renders the city's frightening growth at once marvelous and discrete, figuring metropolitan expansion as a fantastic, but ultimately self-limiting, source of wonder and delight (as a man can grow only so fat, so a city can get only so big). Likewise, to call a man a Lambert of learning is to shape the accomplished mind as a sort of psychological show, to democratize the intellectual heavyweight as a scene of cerebral magnificence whose rarity can be appreciated—if not necessarily achieved—by all. In Daniel Lambert, we can watch one man's fat expand to frame the world. Long after his death, he supplied symbolic largess, his legendary size providing ample coverage for a complex anatomy of uncoordinated cross-references.

Freaks such as Lambert were irreducible at the same time that they

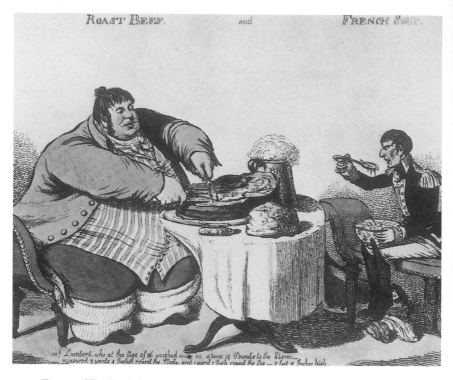

Fig. 31. "The English Lamb and the French Tiger." Engraving by C. W. Williams (1806).

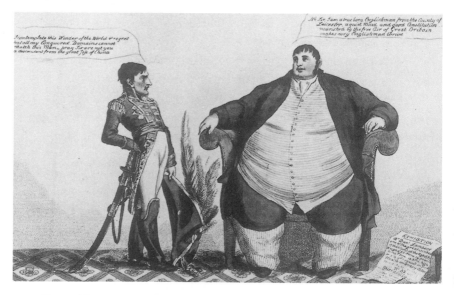

Fig. 32. "Bone and Flesh, or John Bull in Moderate Condition" (1806).

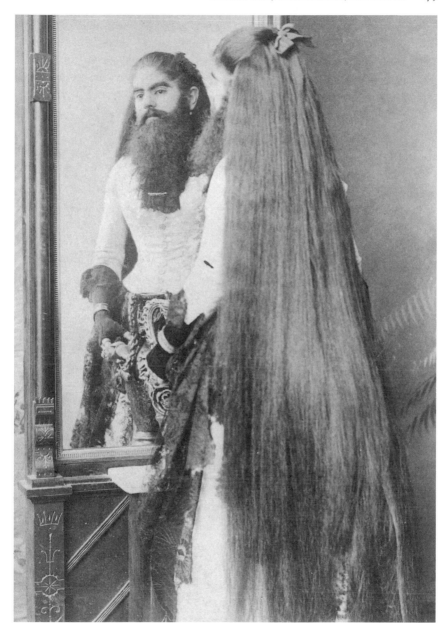

Fig. 33. Annie Jones, one of Barnum's bearded ladies. Photo by Charles Eisenmann, c. 1888. Courtesy of the Becker Collection, Syracuse University, Syracuse, N.Y.

were undecidable: they were definitely indeterminate, determinedly indefinite. Their power lay in their capacity to materialize amorphous symbolic formations, to make the confusion of boundaries devastatingly concrete. Deformity was the stuff of fantasy, a means not of accurately reflecting the world, but of productively distorting it. Like a funhouse mirror, monstrosity was a skewed, skewing lens, a refractory system of significations bent on foiling expectations (fig. 33). In fact, freak shows had nothing to do with realism—even when the monsters they displayed were authentic (and many were not), they were always already fictionalized. With their fake names (Tom Thumb, the Elephant Man, the Sicilian Fairy, the Skeleton Dude) and false histories ("real" and "true" accounts of monsters' lives were full of sensational lies), freaks were lifted into a symbolic structure whose ultimate thrust was to depict the monstrous body as pure representation. Held up for public inspection (fig. 34), freaks were fantastic frames of reference, shocking somatic shorthand for the truth of "normal" existence (Horace Greeley called a pair of microcephalic Salvadoran dwarfs "abridgments, or pocket-editions of Humanity" [quoted in Kunhardt 151]) (fig. 35).

As these examples suggest, the logics I trace in this chapter are not the product of a consistent, clearly articulated series of ideas about either deformity or industrialism; I would be reluctant to describe them as a "rhetoric" or "discourse." Part of what distinguishes them is that they are hardly logical at all. Almost uniformly they are isolated and unmarked; submerged, local, serendipitous, understated, and—like the bodies they exert themselves on—alternately overblown and undeveloped. If monsters were "nature's mistakes," the metaphoric and visual patterns I describe here might be understood as culture's mistakes, the misshapen outgrowths of an ideological system that could not quite contain itself. Monsters worked by implication, by allusion, and, most profoundly, by fallacy—they made sense by not making sense, by meaning in ways that feel far-fetched, inconclusive, accidental, exceptional, and, occasionally, flat-out wrong. Monstrous patterns are in this way ultimately about patterning. They are excessive, disproportionate, odd, and strange; they appear infrequently, at random, and yet are difficult to ignore when they do arise. As such, they call into question the project of cultural criticism itself: to study how the Victorians knew their mon-

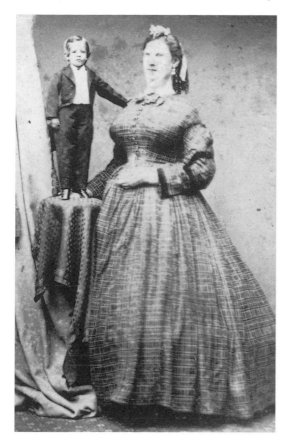

Fig. 34. Anna Swan, one of Barnum's giant-esses, presenting a midget. Courtesy of the Becker Collection, Syracuse University, Syracuse, N.Y.

sters is necessarily to interrogate the terms on which we know—or think we know—the Victorians.

Reading these monstrous moments neither yields a convincing account of how culture works (scattered instants and sheer coincidence cannot sustain the sort of generalizations about ideology or politics that cultural criticism is accustomed to make) nor does it enable a sustained political critique (occasional echoes, overlaps, and chance comparisons can hardly be said to undermine dominant discourses). Rather, reading these monstrous moments might best be understood as an attempt to come to grips with the very questions implied by their status as insufficient evidence—questions having to do with how we write cultural history, with how we accord some patterns political and symbolic centrality and dismiss others as insignificant, flawed, unconvincing, in-

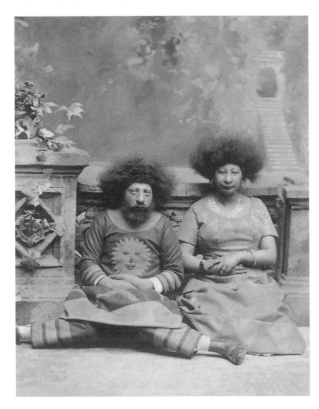

Fig. 35. Maximo and
Bartola, micro-
cephalic Salvadoran
dwarves displayed as
the "Last of the
Ancient Aztecs."
Courtesy of the
Becker Collection,
Syracuse University,
Syracuse N.Y.

complete. Methodologically, then, I am not concerned to construct a
master narrative of Victorian monstrosity, but rather to study what such
a narrative would minimize or even leave out—the linguistic accidents
and visual aberrations that do not add up to much except the sum of a
culture's abortive, aborted, efforts to make meaning. Monsters demonstrate the symbolic utility of conceptual defect. They are ill-conceived
cultural productions whose faulty operations ultimately complicate our
understanding of cultural production as such.

MONSTROUS OBJECTS

Of course, monsters were not the only malformed people running
about Victorian England. As an 1866 article in *Good Words* notes,
"When you come to think of it, we are all of us abnormal, all of us
deformed. Where is the nose that is like the Apollo's, the shoulder that

is like the shoulder of the Milo Venus? Or if we can find perfect single features, where is the artist who has ever seen a perfect 'model'? It may be a new view of the subject to some of us, but we are all of us unquestionably 'deformed,' somewhere or other: in our knees, or our noses, or our finger-ends, or our backs, or our ears, or somewhere else" (Browne 738). Everyone was a little bit off to begin with—and, by the look of things, people were getting worse over time. As countless bluebooks, monographs, and articles argued, city life and labor were taking their toll on the public health. The 1851 census counted 409,207 cases of deformity nationwide and decisively linked urbanization to physical decline: 90,277 (22 percent) of these cases resided in London alone, and the overwhelming bulk of the remaining ones were clustered in England's commercial centers. Bent out of shape by hard work and urban living—"the returns from the manufacturing districts speak of distorted spines as all but universal" ("The Deformed and Their Mental Characteristics" 396)—English subjects seemed to be suffering a massive reformation, a physiological restructuring that coincided with the social restructuring of England itself. As if to say that ill-made physiques are an inevitable by-product of industrialization, the census charts a statistical correlation between manufacture and misshapenness so striking that the one seems to be an index of the other. Cases of arrested development increase in proportion to economic development—"Infirmity of mind and inaptitude to the common offices of life, and undeveloped puberty in both sexes, are constantly reported"—and the result is a nation whose population is as weak as its production is strong: "Out of six hundred and thirteen recruits, only two hundred and thirty-eight were approved for service; the rest were rejected as not strong enough to serve in the defense of their country."

Eighteen fifty-one was, of course, the year of the Great Exhibition, that fabulous monument to progress engineered by Prince Albert and his special Royal Commission. The census was a disturbing subtext to the exhibition's celebration of English commercial success. In calibrating the vexed corporeal status of the people, the census confirmed observations made by Engels, Marx, and others that capitalism was taking place at the expense of the worker's health. More striking, it suggested that capitalism was costing everyone his health, that whether one labored or not, the effect of the factory system was the same:

crooked spines, for example, "were not limited to those who are de-
prived of the comforts of life, for [they were] just as frequent among the
more affluent classes." The census provided hard evidence to support a
growing conviction that bodily degeneration had become the normative condition of industrial modernity.[17] Positing a massive decline in
the physical well-being of the race, theories of degeneration were
deeply concerned with questions of heredity and physical defect; they
read moral and spiritual decay into bodily frailty and used the perceived
increase in deformity to predict racial regression. Degeneration gave a
name and a shape to inchoate anxieties about the underside of industrial development, using deformity as the sign and symptom of a systemic social corruption that far overshadowed the local imperfections
of individual bodies and minds.

Paradoxically, though, the discourse of degeneration theorized the
deformation of Western civilization almost entirely without recourse to
the very bodies that would seem to confirm its claims in no uncertain
terms—the spectacularly misshapen figures of the true terata, the full-
blown monsters that fascinated scientists and spectators alike. With
rare exceptions (Eugene Talbot's *Degeneracy: Its Causes, Signs, and Results* [1898] deserves special note for its frontispiece, a circus photo of
giant and dwarf), the vast literature of degeneration does not interest
itself much in the monster, focusing instead on relatively minor defects
and dysfunctions to make a case for the massive disorder of modern
culture. As a discourse, degeneration performed the anachronistic work
of assimilating the anomaly, absorbing it into an orderly lexicon for
interpreting the steady decomposition of the race. The genealogies of
hereditary decline found in countless studies comprise a remarkably
static catalog of deterioration, their lineages of lapse and loss centering
on a standard series of recurring debasements that together form a
distinctly homogeneous litany of addictions, idiocies, insanities, de-
baucheries, and pathologies:

> An illustration of the variety of stigmata usually to be found among
> the collateral members of a degenerate family is given in the follow-
> ing record: M.D., aged forty-eight, an epileptic during the past two
> years; her father was a drunkard. A sister has a "mother's mark" upon
> the face. A niece has been an epileptic from her twelfth year; her face

is notably asymmetrical, her left ear malformed, there are large "lemurian" outgrowths from her lower jaw, there is a vicious implantation of the lower teeth, she has a right inguinal hernia, a curvature of the spine, and is flat-footed. Another niece has a shaggy "mother's mark" upon the back. M.D. has three children. The eldest, aged nineteen, was backward in learning to walk and talk, he stutters, his lower jaw is poorly developed, his teeth are badly implanted, there is an abnormal projection of the upper dental arch, and the condition of cryptorchidism exists upon the left side. The second child, a daughter, aged seventeen, was backward in walking, and has an umbilical hernia. The third, a boy of eight, had convulsions during the first dentition, and suffers from squint and a congenital fissure of the soft palate. (McKim 90)

Here relative idiosyncrasies become representative pathologies: M.D. and her squinting, seizing, blotchy, botched kin are a model degenerate family. Patterns of decay were so schematic that they could be codified in advance; the alienist Otto Binswanger even drew up a hereditary flow chart:

FIRST GENERATION: Acquired neuropathic condition, drunkenness, dissolute life (acquired moral degeneration).

SECOND GENERATION: Congenital so-called neuropathic constitution, with its concomitant and consequent manifestations (general nervousness, hemicrania, chorea, simple epilepsy, hysteria, and hypochondria).

THIRD GENERATION: Simple primary psychoses (melancholia, mania, paranoia, stuporous insanity, paralysis, etc.), and hysterical and epileptic insanity.

FOURTH GENERATION: "Organically" induced typical forms of hereditary degenerative insanity: periodical and circular insanity, early paranoia, impulsive insanity, sexual perversion, imbecility, and idiocy.

FIFTH GENERATION: Extinction of the thoroughly corrupt family.

(Quoted in McKim 69–70)

Concentrating on a fairly humdrum cluster of disorders, the typical account of degeneration conformed to a predictable taxonomy of both

FAMILY OF A MORAL IMBECILE [1]

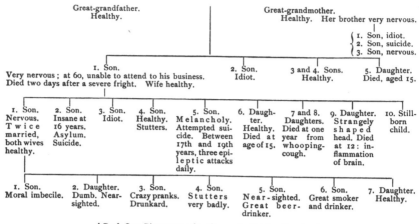

[1] Prof. Otto Binswanger, *loc. cit.*, p. 24, slightly abbreviated.

FAMILY OF THE CRIMINAL SALVATORE MISDEA [1]:

a soldier who, in 1884, by a rapid fusillade, decimated the garrison of his barracks.

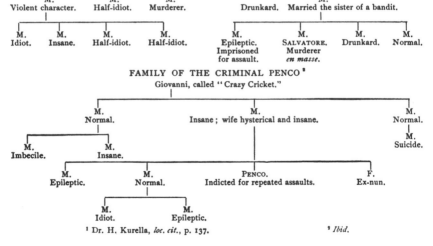

FAMILY OF THE CRIMINAL PENCO [2]

[1] Dr. H. Kurella, *loc. cit.*, p. 137.   [2] *Ibid.*

Fig. 36. Degenerate family trees. From W. Duncan McKim, *Heredity and Human Progress* (1900).

visible and virtual defect, listing aberrations so mundane that one de-generate family tree looks a lot like the next (fig. 36). Rarely is one memorable; seldom can they be told apart. Indeed, their shock value depended in no small degree on the commonness and consistency of familial decline. The narrative of racial decay gained much of its force through the sheer weight of its familiarity—what family didn't number a heavy drinker, a harelip, a hypochondriac, an eccentric aunt, a syphi-litic uncle, or a feeble-minded cousin somewhere in its ranks? Telling the same old story again and again, the discourse of degeneration relied on an increasingly standardized series of somatic signifiers as the stuff of its sensational account of race suicide, discovering doom in the most commonplace anomalies—crossed eyes, a weak chin, attached earlobes, a low forehead—with stunning regularity.

Degeneration was generic. It separated the abnormal from the un-usual, describing a pattern of deviation that ultimately conformed to a narrowly defined pathological norm, a norm that was itself deeply non-descript, an assemblage of interchangeably imperfect parts. As the ty-pological work of men like Galton and Lombroso demonstrated, if you have seen one criminal or prostitute, you have seen them all (fig. 37). Degeneration viewed deformity as practically undetectable, more an indefinite aura than a determined aspect. Robert Louis Stevenson's Mr. Hyde is a classic case: dark, squat, and ugly, he "gives a strong feeling of deformity" although there is "nothing out of the way" (34). Degener-ates ran together, their features blurring into composite types to form a populace whose "impression (from a distance) is of little white blobs of faces borne upon little black twisted or misshapen bodies" (Masterman 121). Degenerates did not stand out in a crowd—they *were* the crowd, a mass of vaguely irregular bodies crushed together to form an unsightly but singularly uniform whole.

The self-proclaimed monsters of the nineteenth century belonged to an entirely different symbolic structure. Monsters were never not a show; they had no anonymity; they were eye-catching, outstanding, absolutely public all the time. The Elephant Man could not leave his home without getting mobbed, and so spent his last days in carefully guarded seclusion. Tom Thumb and his miniature wife, Lavinia, once stopped a funeral procession simply by showing themselves on the street. Drawing crowds wherever they went, monsters stood out in ways

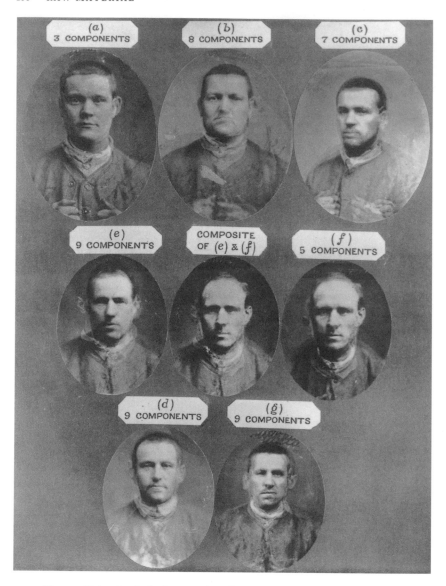

Fig. 37. Galton's criminal composites. From Karl Pearson, *The Life, Letters and Labours of Francis Galton* (1924).

members of the deformed, degenerate public never did. As such, they occupied a bizarre position in relation to the increasingly alienated, alienating mass culture that brought them into being, providing a means of affirming individuality (there was no mistaking a monster) even as they embodied a substantial critique of individuality (no one wanted to *be* a monster).

Where the mild deformations of degeneracy demarcated an undistinguished, indistinctly decaying population, monstrosity was a discourse of uniqueness; indeed, it was in a sense the very sign of individuality. Lewis Carroll articulates this explicitly—if facetiously—in *Through the Looking-Glass* (1872) when Humpty Dumpty tells Alice that she is normal to a fault:

> "Good-bye, till we meet again!" [Alice] said as cheerfully as she could.
>
> "I shouldn't know you again if we *did* meet," Humpty Dumpty replied in a discontented tone, giving her one of his fingers to shake; "you're so exactly like other people."
>
> "The face is what one goes by, generally," Alice remarked in a thoughtful tone.
>
> "That's just what I complain of," said Humpty Dumpty. "Your face is the same as everybody has—the two eyes, so—" (marking their places in the air with his thumb) "nose in the middle, mouth under. It's always the same. Now if you had the two eyes on the same side of the nose, for instance—or the mouth at the top—that would be *some* help."
>
> "It wouldn't look nice," Alice objected. But Humpty Dumpty only shut his eyes, and said, "Wait till you've tried." (135–36)

Freak shows employed a logic very like the one Carroll develops here, celebrating pathological formation as the ultimate mark of personal distinction. Even though there were established types of freaks, every one was billed as one of a kind. Every fat lady was the fattest ever, every dwarf the smallest, every giant the tallest human in history. There were Jane Campbell, "the largest Mountain of Human Flesh ever seen in the form of a woman" (quoted in Saxon 101); and "the Unquestionable Goliath of the Century, CHANG, the CHINESE GIANT, Undoubtedly the Tallest, Largest and Finest Proportioned Giant the Age Has Produced, Standing Nearly 9 Feet High in His Stocking Feet" (quoted in Bogdan 98); and "General Mite! Assuredly the Smallest Man in the World!!" (quoted in Kunhardt 305). Monstrosity shapes a gross anatomy of individuation; as far as the freak show was concerned, anomaly was a superlative achievement, a prodigious feat worthy of admiration and awe.

Where degeneration told a horror story of racial decline, monstrosity was the fairy tale of modern embodiment. The freak show provided an antidote to narratives of hereditary decay, not by disputing the claim that social progress was linked to physical regression, but rather by treating the industrial deformation of the English body as an evolutionarily sound process of adaptation. Certainly, some freaks were framed as throwbacks—after Darwin, there was an endless parade of "missing links," the most famous of whom was Zip, a microcephalic black man whose career spanned the years between 1860 and 1926 (fig. 38).[18] But alongside these timeless characters was a long line of distinctly newfangled figures, monsters made to incarnate distinctly contemporary concerns about what sort of body works best.

In *The Origin of Species* (1859), Darwin defines monsters as contextual creatures: "Monstrosities cannot be separated by any clear line of distinction from mere variations" (72). The difference between the two is one of utility: "By a monstrosity, I presume is meant some considerable deviation of structure in one part, either injurious to or not useful to the species, and not generally propagated" (101). A monstrosity is any mutation without immediate use-value, any genetic anomaly that does not directly enhance an animal's odds of surviving and, of course, reproducing.[19] A variation, by contrast, is potentially adaptive, a trait that does no harm, and might, under the right circumstances, do good. For Darwin, monstrosity and variation are closely linked, mutually constitutive categories, separable only through circumstance. What is beneficial in one situation may be injurious, or monstrous, in another. In evolutionary terms, monstrosity is neither essential nor inherent; it is situational.

Nineteenth-century freak shows developed a selective relativism very like the one we see at work in Darwin, inventing monsters that embodied physiological difference not as degeneration but as pure variation, variation with the potential for seemingly endless innovation

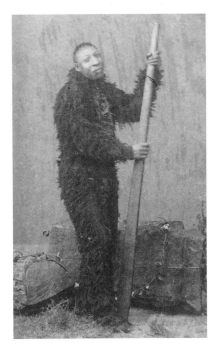 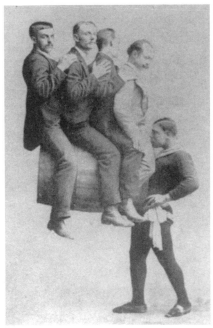

Fig. 38 (left). Zip, one of Barnum's "missing links." Courtesy of the Becker Collection, Syracuse University, Syracuse, N.Y.

Fig. 39 (right). "Iron-Jawed Man." From George M. Gould and Walter L. Pyle, *Anomalies and Curiosities of Medicine* (1901). Courtesy of the College of Physicians, Philadelphia.

and improvement. Ranging their defects as emblems of evolutionary wealth—monsters were the "wonders of God's universe," the richly varied signs of "nature's bounty"—they were, oddly enough, sources of a peculiar brand of hope, an outlandish idealism that situated the monster as the solution to the problem of the social. Monsters adapted themselves to a new species of representation, a high-tech human morphology that extended the promise not of a return to nature, but of nature remade in the image of culture. Holding out the prospect of a corporeality uniquely suited to the particular demands of urban life, monsters shaped a body whose nature it was to merge imperceptibly with culture, a body whose health was constituted as a hybrid blend of human flesh and raw material. There were the iron-jawed men, who could support hundreds of pounds in their teeth (fig. 39); the iron-

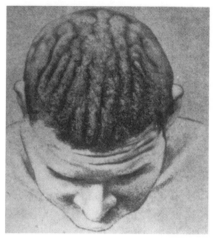
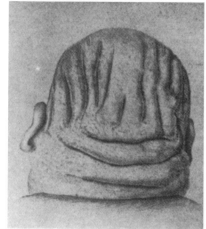

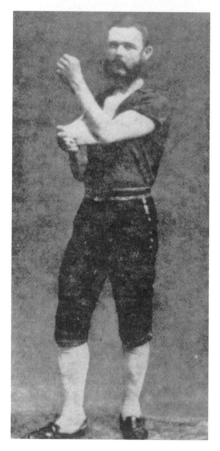

Fig. 40. "Man with Iron Skin."
From George M. Gould and alter L.
Pyle, *Anomalies and Curiosities of
Medicine* (1901). Courtesy of the
College of Physicians, Philadelphia.

Fig. 41. James Morris, one of
Barnum's india-rubber men. From
George M. Gould and Walter L.
Pyle, *Anomalies and Curiosities of
Medicine* (1901). Courtesy of the
College of Physicians, Philadelphia.

skinned men, whose corrugated cuticle was impervious to puncture by knife, dagger, or nail (fig. 40); and the india-rubber men, whose elastic skin stretched far from the body and then snapped back on release, as tight and true as new (fig. 41). There were human magnets so attractive that spoons would adhere to their noses, chins, and fingertips; electric people so vibrant that they gave off sparks (Gould and Pyle 429–30). And there were the fireproof ladies and incombustible men, people who walked on coals, ate fire, and torched themselves to show off flesh that wouldn't burn (fig. 42). Resistant, resilient, and flame-retardant; shock-absorbent, waterproofed, and reinforced; such monsters were walking advertisements for flesh as indestructible quantity. They sold the fiction of an all-purpose, industrial-strength individual: irresistible, enduring, and infinitely cool. The popularity of the freak show may have been a sign of cultural degeneration, but the freaks themselves were, paradoxically, an allegory for the regenerative possibilities contained within the spectacle of decline. Indeed, what the freak show celebrates is a marvelously debased image of industrial existence, a mode of being so phenomenally degraded that it approaches the sublime.

Monstrosity does not register defect as disease; instead, it makes human aberration into an advertisement for a new embodiment. Treating deformity as a healthful adaptation to modern culture, the show celebrates damage as the image of a brave new world. Monsters simultaneously marked the limits of nature, the extent to which a body could deviate from fixed norms of health and still live, and the end of culture, the point beyond which the transformative powers of human industry could not go (freaks were beyond the curative powers of science). As such, they imaged a weird amalgam of nature and culture, an amazing biotechnology in which the birth defect framed a varied and expansive commentary on consumer culture's material distortions—to bodies, to goods, and to representations.

Susan Stewart has observed that a period's freaks expose its particular standardizations (133). The Victorian freak exhibits a curiosity about standardization itself, entertaining the anachronistic notion that reducing the body to a mechanical prototype could be the very condition of selfhood rather than the means of taking it away. We can see this in the model of individualism promoted by the sideshow. By definition, every

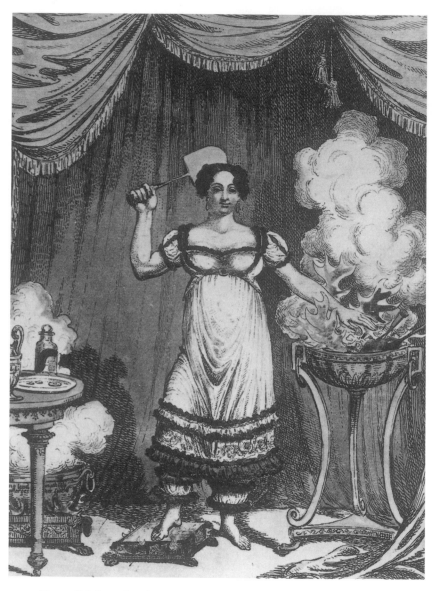

Fig. 42. Madame Giradelli, the Celebrated Fire Proof Female. Engraving by C. W. Williams (c. 1818).

monster was one of a kind. But monsters themselves were a dime a dozen. Every show had the fattest woman on earth and the skinniest man; every show featured a bearded lady, a giant, a dwarf, and an albino family. With the exception of celebrities such as Tom Thumb, these figures were infinitely renewable—the names and faces changed over time, but the basic configuration of the show remained the same. The result was a sort of assembly-line individualism, an endless procession of human oddities whose cumulative impact was to standardize abnormality itself, to reduce the scene of nature's bounty to a series of predictable, replaceable originals.

It is not surprising, then, that questions of utility, efficiency, work, and waste—of effort, energy, and motion—are never far from monsters. Most monsters became monsters, after all, because they could not do traditional forms of work. And the terms on which monsters were displayed presupposed a basic analogy between physical malfunction and mechanical operation, an alignment that manifested itself most often as an abiding interest in what freaks could do. For example, Barnum found his Highland fat boys less interesting as fat boys than as examples of fat in action: "The Scotch boys were interesting, not so much on account of their weight, as for the mysterious method by which one of them, though blindfolded, answered questions put by the other respecting objects presented by spectators" (Barnum 346–47). Similarly, what made armless and legless wonders wonderful was their ability to perform operations normally done by the missing limbs: writing with toes, walking on hands, or serving tea and knitting with feet were all part of the limbless stock in trade. Monsters neutralized the notion of incapacity, transforming gross defect into rare skill and making even serious injury look like nothing: Charles Warren made a name for himself in both medical and show circles as a "dislocationist" by throwing his bones far out of joint and then replacing them at will (Gould and Pyle 473–74). Exhibiting a profound physiological resourcefulness, monsters made spectacles of their own extraordinary powers of compensation. Making the most of what they had (as Tom Thumb put it, "I feel as big as anybody"), monsters made a virtue—and sometimes a fortune—of necessity. In the process they redefined necessity itself: after all, the scene of an ill-made body making do was always on some level a perverse promotion for what a body could do without.

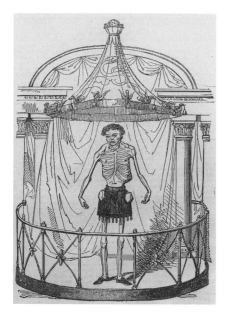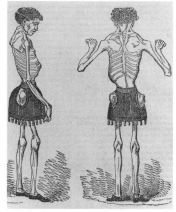

Fig. 43. Claude Ambroise Seurat, the Living Skeleton. From William Hone, *The Every-day Book and Table Book* (1837–38).

Take flesh. Living skeletons were less noteworthy for having no meat on their bones than for not needing any. As one observer wrote of Claude Seurat, a French skeleton who showed himself during the early decades of the nineteenth century, "the curiosity, as it really exists, lies far less in the degree of attenuation which Seurat's frame exhibits, than in the fact that, with a frame so reduced, a human being should be still in possession of most of his functions, and enjoying a reasonable quantity of health. As regards the exhibition of bone, for instance, there is not so much as may frequently be found (in the dead subject) in cases where persons have died of lingering consumption" (Hone 1027) (fig. 43). Seurat was remarkable for looking like he was starving to death when he was really quite well. So was Isaac Sprague, who showed off his virility by being photographed with his well-fed wife and three sturdy little boys (fig. 44). Unlike the diseased, the dying, and the malnourished poor, living skeletons appeared to thrive without flesh: in the process, they made deprivation itself seem insubstantial.

Arms were as inessential as flesh. Without arms, one is without

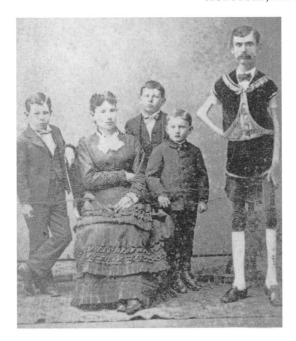

Fig. 44. Isaac Sprague and family. Courtesy of the Becker Collection, Syracuse University, Syracuse, N.Y.

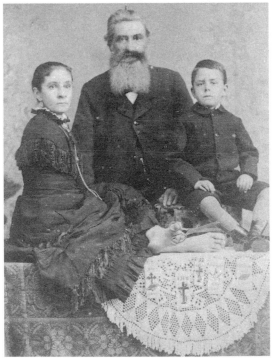

Fig. 45. Ann Leak Thompson. Courtesy of the Becker Collection, Syracuse University, Syracuse, N.Y.

hands; armlessness reduces reach and dismembers dexterity. The armless wonder disproved this seemingly straightforward premise, making up for missing limbs by using legs, feet, and toes to perform all the tasks typically done with arms and hands—eating, writing, shaving, smoking, sewing, painting, knitting, whittling, and even playing musical instruments. Sanders Nellis, a Barnum regular, cut out Valentines, wound his watch, loaded and fired a pistol, and shot a bow and arrow, all with his feet. Ann Leak Thompson was an exceptionally pious woman who worked religious symbols into her crocheting and embroidery (fig. 45). And the famous Charles Tripp spent upward of fifty years doing carpentry, painting portraits, and practicing penmanship before appreciative audiences (fig. 46). The ultimate thesis of the armless act is that arms aren't really necessary after all; as Ann Leak Thompson liked to write, "So you perceive it's really true, when hands are lacking, toes will do" (quoted in Bogdan 217). Armless wonders were monuments to ingenuity, discipline, and hard work. Able to perform "many . . . things with his feet, which a vast majority of mankind cannot with their hands," Sanders Nellis was billed as "an instance of what can be accomplished by a strong mind, aided by indomitable perseverance and untiring industry" (quoted in Bogdan 216).

Staging the peculiar efficacy of the body with no hands, armless wonders were the symbolic counterpart to that other well-known image of disarticulated efficiency, the factory "hand." The problem with the industrial hand was that it had a body—as Dickens put it, "hands" were "a race who would have found more favor with some people if Providence had seen fit to make them only hands, or, like the lower creatures of the seashore, only hands and stomachs" (*Hard Times* 70). And the problem with the hand's hands was that they were always in danger of getting mangled, or even cut off. According to Engels, the most common factory accident was "the squeezing off of a single joint of a finger, somewhat less common the loss of the whole finger, half or a whole hand, an arm, etc., in the machinery." Such injuries had "for the operative the secondary effect of unfitting him for his work more or less completely" (173). Installing a split between the presence of defect and the state of being defective, the armless wonder made physical deficiency the condition for an exemplary mechanical efficiency. The image

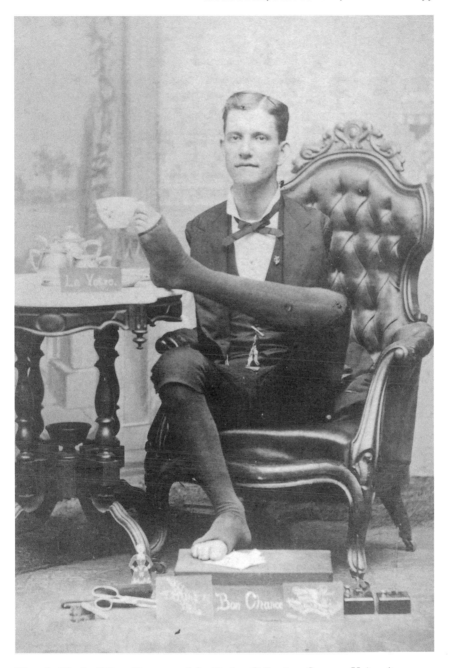

Fig. 46. Charles Tripp. Courtesy of the Becker Collection, Syracuse University, Syracuse, N.Y.

of a dismembered dexterity, the armless wonder sidestepped the problem instantiated in the factory "hand" simply by doing without. As far as the sideshow is concerned, the answer to the laboring hand with a body is a clever body with no hands. In the sideshow, conceptual sleight of hand recuperates the industrial accident as the very image of evolutionary fitness, creating an individual so capable of capitalizing on his deficiencies that he can embrace (if only with his legs) a lifestyle that would otherwise be beyond his reach. Portraits bear witness to this, showing wonders as unexceptional members of respectable families.

Like the prosthetic man, the armless wonder embodies a fantasy of social mobility. Both represent the power of discipline to secure a desirable standard of living for the physically compromised subject; both imagine disability away, treating mutilation and deformity as conditions that can be overcome by dint of hard work and strength of character. They differ fundamentally, however, in their mode of imagining. The discourse of prosthesis fetishizes the body so perfectly rebuilt that the fact of limb loss can go virtually undetected. By contrast, the freak show celebrates the absence of prosthesis (not to mention reduction, correction, and cure), instead idealizing anomaly as the very sign of social well-being.[20] Where prosthetics model a more perfect flesh, the armless wonder exemplifies the ideal machine.

The fantasy of physical reduction as a mode of heightened mechanical efficiency reaches its apotheosis in Henry Ford's description of his ideal factory as an assembly line manned by strategically dis-assembled workers. In his 1922 autobiography, Ford notes that 7,882 separate work operations were required to make the model T—but that only 12 percent (949) of them needed "strong, able-bodied, and practically physically perfect men." Of the rest, "we found that 670 could be filled by legless men, 2,637 by one-legged men, 2 by armless men, 715 by one-armed men, and 10 by blind men" (108–9). Imaging systematic deformation as the condition of production, Ford uses deformity to contemplate the prospect of a perfectly streamlined body, one as compact and purposeful as machinery itself. Indeed, one might argue that Ford imagines the deformed body *as* the perfectly streamlined body. The whole body—normally the quintessential sign of personal and social well-being—stands here *in absentia* as a sort of luxury model, a form of excess, a waste of flesh. Mark Seltzer reads this passage as a paean to prosthesis, an industrial dream in which man and machine meet, merge, and complete one another (*Bodies and Machines* 157). Such a reading depends on a purely metaphoric model of prosthesis, however, and seems to me to cover up the strikingly literal nature of Ford's point—that uncorrected amputations, mutilations, and aberrations are the raw material of an ideal industrial world; that they enable the ultimate division of labor, bodies reduced to the bare essentials of perfectly executed work operations. Ford's is not so much a fantasy of prosthesis, of building an incomplete body up, as one of partitioning, of paring the body down. The ideal here is physique as pure framework: no extras, bare bones, minimal, minimized; only what is needed to work. This is the Victorian image of the disembodied factory hand pushed to its furthest extreme, the progressive reduction of the natural body as a technical adjustment, a strategic upgrade that yields an ideal—even utopian—state of productivity. Growing out of logics launched during the nineteenth century, Ford's fantasy makes explicit what is everywhere implied by Victorian deployments of deformity: that the mechanically impaired body might be the body most perfectly suited to a culture of machines. In the nineteenth-century sideshow, we see the body with fewer parts becoming the ultimate tool. Treating anatomical downsizing as mechanical upgrade, the sideshow acts by imaginative proxy, employing the armless wonder as a fantastic hand.

Arms as options, expendable accessories—it was a gripping idea. The Victorian sideshow played with arms in their absence, made them into detachable parts, extensions a body could well do without. Such symbology had its limits, however. Barnum was happy to display bodies without arms, but he couldn't stomach the idea of displaying a telephone—a contraption he viewed as an arm without a body (Ronell 301). Barnum worried that the telephone was a greater curiosity than his freaks and would be more than his public could handle. Strange, considering how closely aligned the monster was with the mechanical oddity. After all, Barnum himself made monsters into metonymical gizmos. So did Twain, who wrote about conjoined twins as a fabulously efficient gimcrack, a "pair of scissors" (*Pudd'nhead Wilson* 267), or "one of those pocket-knives with a multiplicity of blades" (244) whose weird,

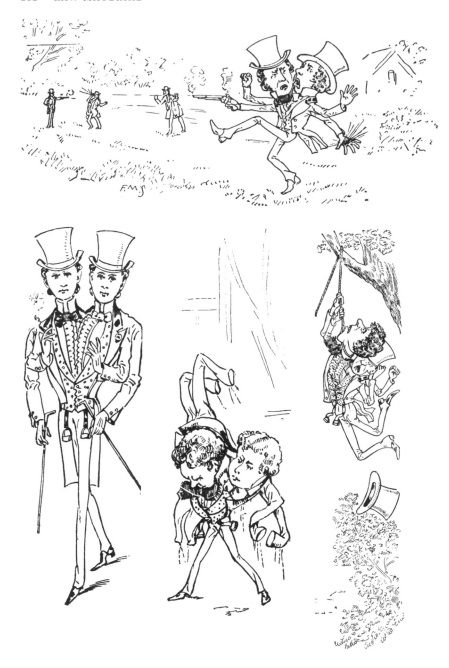

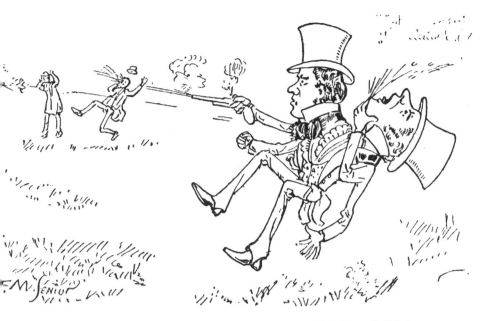

Fig. 47 (above and opposite). Siamese gadget. Illustrations by F. M. Senior for Mark Twain, *Those Extraordinary Twins* (1894).

complicated workings were a "great economy" that "saves time and labor" (246) (fig. 47). Twain's imagery recalls one of the more outstanding appliances displayed at that fabulous showcase for arcane invention, the Crystal Palace. There, amid collapsible pianos (for playing on yachts), defensive locks that shot at anyone who tried to pick them, marble-topped ornamental stoves, papier-mâché furniture, hot-air balloons, sewing machines, rubber clothing, and artificial limbs, stood a gorgeously overwrought knife boasting more than eighty different blades: sort of a sharper image of Twain's twin blades (fig. 48). Monster as gadget, gadget as monster: each invoked the other. These associations make a certain amount of sense: monsters and gadgets each labored under essentially the same functional problem. Monsters were too oddly formed to work in the real world, and gadgets were often so strangely contrived that they just didn't work—the baroque knife's special qualification, for instance, was that it was too specialized to be used. In a world obsessed with maximizing productivity, both monsters and gadgets occupied the liminal, compromised position of the potentially

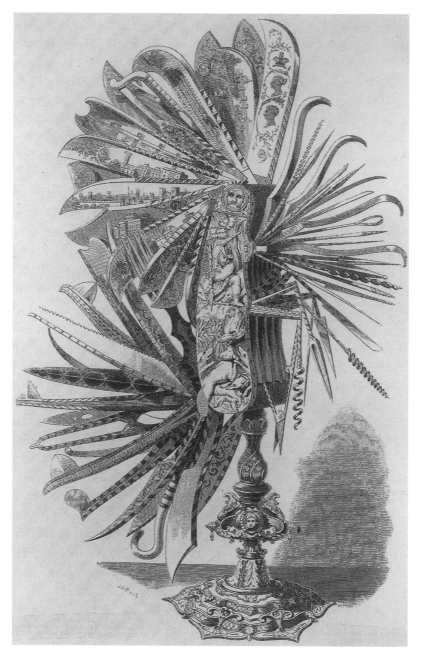

Fig. 48. Overwrought knife. From *The Official Descriptive and Illustrated Catalogue of the Great Exhibition of the Works of Industry of All Nations, 1851* (1851).

useless object. So it is that the laborious allusions of sideshows and side notes broke down into oddly unworkable figures for each other.

Household Words engineered yet another in this running series of incompetent images when it made an elaborately confusing analogy between a dismantled sewing machine and Sarah Biffin, one of the most famous limbless women of the century. Describing the sewing machine as an "iron seamstress," the essay recounts a battle between two competing inventors for patent rights to some of her more intricate parts:

> Part of the iron lady (said Mr. Howe) might belong to Mr. Judkins; but, undoubtedly, the lady's hands—the needle and the shuttle— were the property of Mr. Howe. Howe versus Judkins hereupon joined issue, and the law decided in favor of Howe. What does the seamstress then, but appear, like Miss Biffin, without arms! These were terrible times in the history of the metallic seamstress. But Mr. Judkins did not desert the lady in these her dark days. He forthwith proceeded to consider the possibility of adapting the seamstress to her work. He succeeded. She now proceeds to do her business in a curious, but effective way. She is, probably, not good at involved crochet-patterns, and in other mysteries of needlework; but give her plain work to sew, and you shall see her make more than five hundred tight stitches in a minute.
>
> The iron seamstress is composed of a flat metal surface, about twelve inches square (a very comfortable little body, as it will be seen), resting on four substantial legs. From one side of the lady's flat iron surface, an arm rises to the height of about ten inches, and then, bending the elbow, passes over to the opposite side. From the end of the arm, a moveable finger descends; this moveable finger holds the needle. But, the iron lady's needle is not like the instrument of a flesh and blood seamstress. Her needle has its eye only half an inch from the point. (Jerrold 576)

Hardly a seamless comparison: sewing machine amputated into armless wonder, armless wonder built into sewing machine with an artificial limb, artificial limb made in the image of a sewing machine's arm. This is a metaphor that works by hemming itself in, ending in a needle

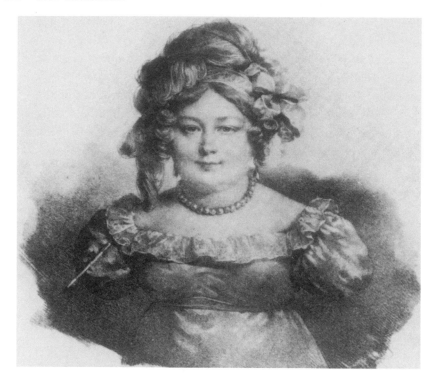

Fig. 49. Miss Biffin. Lithograph (1823) courtesy of Ricky Jay.

whose singular efficiency is always already beside the point: the real Miss Biffin remained uncorrected and made a living painting porcelain with a brush held in her mouth (figs. 49, 50).

True to the logic of carnival, freak shows celebrated an image of the social that was elsewhere seen as profoundly threatening.[21] Where social critics loudly bemoaned the debasement of taste and manners that seemed to attend the rise of the mass market, freak shows sold the dissolution of culture as cheap amusement, lauding the loss of distinction as the stuff of laughter. And while fears of racial decline spurred the development of social Darwinist programs such as eugenics, the freak show applauded physical degeneration, using it to stage a kind of inverted eugenics, a skewed social vision in which gross deformity contained the promise of a regenerative body politics. Taking destruction by disease as a strategic reconstruction of the body, the freak show rebuilt the self as object. In thus refracting the monster through the lens of

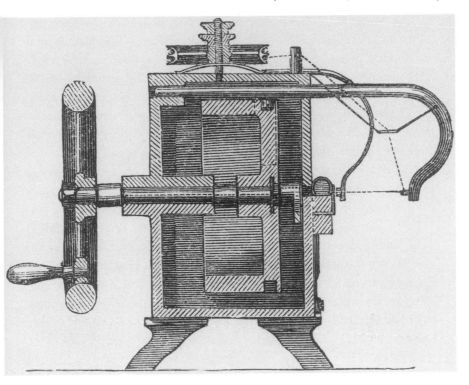

Fig. 50. The iron seamstress. From *The Official Descriptive and Illustrated Catalogue of the Great Exhibition of the Works of Industry of All Nations, 1851* (1851).

material culture by likening the deformed body to unusual things, the freak show framed the quintessential nightmare of capitalism—total objectification—as a viable mode of being. In this way, the freak show stood as a carnivalesque counterpoint to emergent theories of economic oppression. While social critics were developing theories of oppression that centered on the objectifying effects of machine work, monsters opened up a space in which to consider objectification not as a dehumanizing process, as Marx would have it, but rather as a potentially adaptive response to a culture increasingly organized around the production and consumption of goods. Imagining the self as an evacuated, eviscerated surface of distorted efficiency, the freak show proposed the bad dream of automation as a technique of individuation, a devolutionary strategy for producing a more fit—and fitting—humanity.

In so doing, monsters incarnated a distinctly vulgar mode of imagining. Freaks embodied the conceptual utility of vulgarity (not to mention the vulgarity of utility), incorporating a logic whereby monstrous analogy, gross generalization, and distorted perception could seem rational and even natural. Soliciting twisted logic and truncated reasoning, deformity was a means of making imperfect associations across disparate discursive and social spaces, and so of generating new bodies of knowledge (however badly formed). Deformity disorganized definitions, destabilizing notions of the natural (human wonders marked the extreme limits of life), and in the process producing a warped way of seeing the social, an epistemology that collapsed pathology and progress so totally that monstrous people became perverse parables of culture. Victorian monsters were all-purpose symbolic devices, capable of standing for everything from the machines flooding the marketplace to the marketplace itself. Perhaps it was with this in mind that in 1853, one enterprising giant advertised himself as "the true Great Exhibition" (Wood 222). Freak shows were above all comedies of objectification, hysterical send-ups of a marketplace that was taking people for all they were worth.

The Promises of Monsters, or,
A Manifesto for Academic Futures

Deformito-mania did not die out with the Victorians. Indeed, the hunger for monstrosity is alive and well in late twentieth-century culture. There are the monster movies, the freakish personalities (Michael Jackson once tried to cement his affinity with monstrosity by purchasing the Elephant Man's bones), the talk shows (often called freak shows) with their endless parade of perversities. Deformity is the stuff of art as well as popular entertainment; witness the photography of Diane Arbus and Joel-Peter Witkin, or novels such as Katherine Dunn's *Geek Love,* Ursula Hegi's *Stones from the River,* John Irving's *Son of the Circus,* and Elizabeth McCracken's *The Giant's House.* So expansive is contemporary deformito-mania that even cultural criticism has yielded to its influence. Consider the recent flood of scholarly books, chapters, articles, and anthologies on the subject of deformity. There are literary and cultural histories on everything from *Frankenstein* to bodybuilding; sociological studies of disability; psychoanalytic, feminist, postcolonial, and narrative theories of what monsters mean, how they are made, what they can tell us about the mind, the body, language, and power.[1] There is a monster for every occasion and an occasion for every conceivable kind of monster. Taken in its unwieldy entirety, "monster theory," as one collection calls it, has evolved into one of the signature subfields of contemporary cultural theory. If the Victorians suffered from a passion for freaks so severe that it was diagnosed, however playfully, as a new form of social madness, contemporary criticism evinces such an abiding fascination with the history and theory of monsters that it too might be said to labor under an abnormal preoccupation.

We don't have to look far to understand the intellectual fashion for deformity, for critical monsters work much as more popular ones do: in theory as in life (monsters demand such stagy contrasts), monsters are remarkably demonstrative subjects, the spectacular arbiters of social and political tastes. Just as nineteenth-century freak shows celebrated liberal ideals of self-determination in the shape of the well-adjusted human wonder, contemporary cultural criticism places the monster at the center of its effort to reimagine the power relations that mediate and all too often determine the limits of human possibility. Forming the centerpiece of studies on issues as varied as reproduction, imperialism, creativity, carnival, spectacle, and the rise of mass culture, monsters seem not only to be everywhere, but also to be able to mean just about anything. Whatever the context, though, the "monster" is a figure for what is transgressive and liminal; as we have seen, a monster by definition describes the simultaneous violation of physical and metaphysical boundaries. Psychoanalytic approaches, for example, see the monster as an articulation of the edges of humanness, a dramatic vision of what separates self and other at both collective and individual levels.[2] Postcolonial critiques focus on the prevalence of nonwhite people in the sideshow, arguing that the representation of perfectly healthy racial and ethnic others as monsters provided an imaginative rationale for the racist and imperialist practices that have characterized recent Western history.[3] Since the 1970s, feminist criticism has noted the historic monstrousness of any female body, deformed or not.[4] Most recently, the exhibition of "human oddities" has been described as a disturbing chapter in the history of the disabled.[5] However they are presented, monsters reveal monstrous aspects of human relations; and they do so both over time (in the history of Western exploitation) and out of it (in the depths of a psyche whose nature it is to understand itself over and against its others). Patrick Brantlinger has written that the main "lesson" cultural studies offers is that "in order to understand ourselves, the discourse of 'the Other'—of all the Others—is that which we most urgently need to hear" (3). As the consummate Other, a body whose spectacular deviations work to clarify the limits of what is considered to be normal, the monster is uniquely suited to facilitate the ongoing analysis of power, representation, and subject formation that characterizes so much of contemporary academic writing. In so doing, it both facilitates analysis of the very sorts of oppression it originally helped to consolidate, and continues to function in its Victorian guise, as a means of mobilizing new perspectives on culture.

For the extent to which monsters enable us to do cultural theory is the extent to which we are still—for all our postmodern machinations— eminently Victorian. Despite the obvious historical, political, and cultural differences separating the nineteenth-century freak show from contemporary cultural studies, the two share a fundamental similarity of tone, topic, and intent. Both rely on the attraction of atypical and even distasteful subject matter to lure an audience. And both see that questionable attraction as essentially teachable (not to mention profitable); each imagines its audience as a malleable public, as something that can be educated and enlightened—about politics, scholarship, identity, anatomy, the world—even as it is being entertained. Although the one sees itself as an integral part of a budding mass culture while the other seeks to critique the very concept of mass culture, the two share a common representational structure and a related series of imaginative goals. They even show a similar ambivalence toward their own shock value, going to great (if necessarily ineffectual) lengths to control the type of emotion they elicit. As we have seen, the Victorian freak show frequently managed monstrosity's effects by casting the monster as not shocking—as an essentially normal person capable of work, play, and love. Contemporary cultural studies, by contrast, contains its monsters by a strategic displacement: what is shocking is not deformity itself (which sensitivity training enjoins us not to notice fully), but how deformity has historically been exploited, displayed for what Robert Bogdan so concisely calls "amusement and profit." Where the Victorian freak show claimed to exploit the moral and educational potential of prurient interest as such (staring at the monster will eventually bring a person into focus), today the proper affective relation to the freak show is moral outrage (more than any other scene of objectification, the freak show makes visible the dehumanizing power of the gaze). In its seemingly inexhaustible desire to display and dissect the politics of defor-

mity, cultural studies is a freak show—albeit a studiously correct one—
in its own right. (The recent popularity of carnival as a rubric for
thinking culture serves as a tacit acknowledgment of this fact: what else
is the critic, in this context, but a consummate showman?)[6]

I draw this parallel between the display tactics of the Victorian freak
show and the analytical procedures of cultural studies with caution—
my wish is neither to disregard the very real distinctions that are there
to be made between the Victorians' penchant for exhibiting human
wonders and contemporary scholarship's attraction to unusual and unsettling subjects nor to denigrate cultural studies by identifying it as a
form of the exploitation it seeks to critique. Rather, my interest lies in
the substantial utility of such an openly vulgar comparison. For bringing two such antithetical institutions into alignment allows each to
illuminate the other in subtle, surprising ways. Cultural studies has
made monsters newly visible, and monsters themselves lie at the heart
of cultural studies, helping to frame its mission and even giving shape to
its projected future. So pervasive are monsters, and so consistent is their
attachment to issues dear to cultural studies's resolutely topical, political heart, that it is tempting to see their popularity as a result of their
conceptual utility: to see, in other words, criticism's deformito-mania as
a symptom of its ongoing struggle for self-definition. Like the Victorian syndrome that preceded it, this deformito-mania is a profoundly
useful obsession for a field in a disturbing state of flux, one that provides
a focal point for thinking through the question of what criticism can
and should be.

Recent work on monsters argues that monsters are, above all, made
entities, telling products of their time. Embodying the anxieties and
exhilarations of the moment in which they are born, they are ciphers for
culture, misshapen blank slates who tell us everything about their world
while revealing next to nothing about themselves. Read in this light,
critical monsters behave just as one would expect, providing telling
insight into the political, conceptual, and emotional terms on which
contemporary scholarship is founded. It strikes me as no accident that
monster studies has emerged at a moment of professional identity crisis, a moment when it is no longer clear to us exactly who we are, what
we do, and whether we matter to the world at large. Anxieties about the
social relevance, intellectual mission, and institutional well-being of

criticism are running so high that an entire genre of scholarly writing has emerged to address the practical and philosophical issues that are being raised by the current crisis in the humanities.[7] The monster sits at the center of contemporary debates about the social utility of academic work. As a major figure in recent cultural critique, the monster has been an exemplary subject through which to display the radical social consciousness of political criticism. It has also supplied an enormously helpful vocabulary for thinking about the shape of criticism itself.

Donna Haraway's "Promises of Monsters: A Regenerative Politics for Inappropriate/d Others" stands as the most dramatic instance of such anomalous self-fashioning. This seminal essay in the field of cultural studies appeared in the landmark volume *Cultural Studies* and is itself a *monstre par excès*, a futuristic philosophical dream in which a metaphoric "womb of a pregnant monster" carries the theoretical possibility of rescuing the planet from "the amniotic effluvia of terminal industrialism" (295–96). As such, Haraway's essay draws on the monster's historical association with transgressive alterity in order to articulate a passionately hopeful vision of change. For Haraway, the monster embodies the transformative potential of a cultural theory truly capable of thinking beyond categorical constraint; it is a symbol of a utopian future born of a genuinely effective political criticism. More recently, though, the monster has become a prominent figure in comparatively depressed thinking about the state of the profession. Bruce Robbins has analyzed how the university's professionalization of the intellectual has created a "monster to be repudiated and ridiculed" by both left and right (4). Patricia Meyer Spacks has commented on how an exaggerated preprofessionalism has resulted in a "deformation" of graduate studies (quoted in Guillory 92). And John Guillory has described the academic job market as a "monstrous contingency," arguing that "graduate students are condemned to suffer most from the symptoms of a pathology that afflicts the profession universally" (93–94). Since Haraway published her promising conception in 1992, monsters have come to stand for the very forms of institutional stasis they were originally seen to resist. It is as if the monster's power to shape desirable changes has weakened with age, has degenerated into a cipher for the degeneration of the profession itself. So it is that Robert Miklitsch's letter in *PMLA*'s 1997 forum on cultural studies's relation to the literary launches its claims by casting out the monster: "Cultural studies is not some Frankensteinian monster come to vanquish literature (unless, of course, one reads Frankenstein as the return of the mass-cultural repressed and literature as the embodiment of classical bourgeois culture). Rather, cultural studies, as intellectually partisan and methodologically motley as it sometimes is, should be considered part of a larger process of regeneration, where regeneration for both literature and cultural studies is only possible when there is a thorough acknowledgment of the past as well as the present future" (258). With its emphasis on the "regenerations" enabled by an avowedly "utopian" (258) approach to textual study, the passage echoes Haraway's concept of a regenerative criticism. The difference is that where Haraway sees the monster as the symbol of theoretical rebirth, Miklitsch depicts the monster as the sterile, sterilizing enemy of an academic revitalization enabled by a cultural studies that is both passably mainstream (not some monster) and so radically "motley" that even the image of alterity itself, the monster, cannot properly contain it. Finer points of usage aside, the bigger picture here is clear enough: whether casting the monster as an enemy of criticism or embracing it as a metaphor for transformative critique, the cultural theory of the 1990s used the idea of the monster to focus its own political vision.

Such an anatomy of reference is hardly surprising when we consider that the professional anxiety monsters most immediately express is an anxiety of extinction. On the one hand, academics labor increasingly under a debilitating fear that genuinely searching academic work is fast becoming a vestigial structure, a useless and hence expendable appendage to a culture that neither values nor understands it. On the other hand, current trends in scholarship seem to many to endanger the well-being of disciplines from within. This danger is felt, ironically, at precisely the point at which so much recent academic work seeks to answer the charge that it is not properly grounded in reality: cultural studies. Born out of a pressing need to frame historical and textual analyses as important actors in the world outside the university, contemporary cultural studies (along with its more formal parent, new historicism) seeks to establish criticism as a radical and necessary form of activism. But in its unorthodox choice of material and its resolutely underspecified methodology, cultural studies has posed a substantial threat to the future of the disciplines even as it has breathed new life and purpose into academic work.[8] In the case of English, the discipline from within which this book was written, this anxiety manifests itself as a fear for the future of literary study—which cultural studies includes but does not privilege—and, more basically, for the future of textual analysis (as literature disappears, the argument goes, close reading will be lost along with it).[9] Criticism's monsters embody the tensions of a particularly fraught professional moment, at once announcing the power of intellectual work to participate in the creation of a better world and articulating concomitant anxieties that criticism as we know it is dying out. As such, they indicate the extent to which criticism's choice of language and subject matter are embedded in an ongoing effort to understand what criticism actually is—what it can do, what it has done, what it might become. As both a topic and a recurring metaphor, the monster tells us as much about the intellectual climate of the present moment as it does about past structures of thought.

In more ways than one, then, monsters have given the profession a chance to reflect—to theorize the body as the place where power has historically assumed its most monstrous and its most liberatory incarnations, and to think passionately, obsessively, sometimes even manically about what it means to do criticism itself. And in this sense, the questions monsters raise regarding the politics of critical attention are central to this book. My own interest in monsters lies in their historical tendency to offer up a sort of embodied cultural theory, a theory that has, since at least the nineteenth century, centered increasingly on the tense relation between the perceived impropriety of freak shows and the very real conceptual utility of shocking display. That interest in turn has modulated the whole of *Raw Material*, whose own shocking displays (of which monsters are, ironically, the least unsettling) have been rendered with an eye toward forcing the complex and troubling connections between historical patterns and critical paradigms into view. For if one of my most pressing aims is to insist on the deep, total entanglement of the raw materials of history and the methods cultural critics use for studying and writing about that history, my central tactic has been to bring the close-reading skills usually associated with English departments to bear on material that seems initially to be ill suited to the sorts of interpretive play that a rapt attention to language renders inevitable. It is the discomfiting, even unnerving clash between sensitive subject matter and sensitive reading that has interested me most here: if *Raw Material* has done its work, it has subjected both "the body" (whose analytical power has been weakened by overexposure) and cultural studies (which has yet to uncover the full extent of its own analytical investments) to a necessary defamiliarization. And in so doing, it has not only yielded new arguments about the place of "the body" in Victorian self-fashioning, but has understood those arguments as efforts to work through some of the fraught connections among English (whose attachment to literature makes it reluctant to see its practitioners turn their attention to other sorts of texts), historiography (which, despite the much-debated "linguistic turn," still tends to regard the close reading of nonliterary texts with suspicion), interdisciplinarity (which tends not to respect, or even fully to grasp, the special techniques of disciplines), and that vague but powerful category that looms in the background of these border wars and animates work like *Raw Material:* cultural studies.

This book is about what happens to reading in a nonliterary context; about what happens to history when nonliterary texts (the raw materials of historical analysis) are subjected to sustained, creative close reading; and about what happens to method when it is read as a part of the history it is helping to write. As such, it is above all an argument for close reading, particularly for close reading beyond the boundaries of the literary text—not in order to distort "history" by treating it as an infinitely flexible narrative, nor to write a more "truthful" history by framing new master narratives, but, rather, to insist on the capacity of close reading to reveal precisely those moments when the competing prerogatives of textual analysis and contextual fidelity come into contact. The use of "literary" devices such as metaphor, synecdoche, and analogy in nonfictional spaces has thus been a central focus of this book, a means of charting conceptual links both within Victorian culture and, perhaps most strikingly, between past discursive formations and present strategies for revealing and resisting them. In the last analysis, then, we might most properly describe *Raw Material* as a book about contemporary critical practice, a book whose particular focus on Victorian culture provides the basis for a study of how we study culture. In attempting to uncover Victorian logics of signification, this volume finally asks a far more elemental and ultimately elusive set of questions about how our own analytical styles and political projects work to make the past signify, significant. In this it is itself a hopeful monster, a sustained attempt to conceive a criticism whose disturbances contain the germ of something strangely useful and new.

INTRODUCTION

1 Of course, political analogies between the body and the social system have existed for centuries. This book concerns itself with the uniquely Victorian dimensions of this figure, analyzing how literal and figurative links between disease and modernization affected Victorian notions of embodiment. Constituted as a response to the material conditions of towns, the Victorian social body provided a shorthand for talking about the effects of urbanization and industrialization on national well-being. Implicitly poor, unwashed, urban, and unwell, the social body was framed as a collective entity whose signature feature was its absolute vulnerability to the living conditions produced by modern urban life. See Mary Poovey's *Making a Social Body: British Cultural Formation, 1830–1864* for an analysis of how the conceptual shift from "body politic" to "social body" turned on an increasing awareness, from the 1830s on, of the damaging effects of urbanization on human life. See also Catherine Gallagher's essay "The Body versus the Social Body in the Works of Thomas Malthus and Henry Mayhew."

2 Tuberculosis caused around one-third of all deaths between 1800 and 1850; its mortality was halved between 1850 and 1910. Even so, it remained the most significant cause of death after heart disease, and as late as the 1890s tuberculosis was estimated to kill three times more people every year than the Crimean War had (Wohl 130). Historians conjecture that the decline in the disease after midcentury was less a consequence of improved living conditions than the result of the gradual waning common to virulent contagious disease over time. Statistics on tuberculosis during this period are necessarily vague—until Koch isolated the tuberculosis bacillus in 1882, the disease was frequently confused with other wasting diseases such as cancer. Nevertheless, the distinctive symptoms of tuberculosis—the hacking cough, the hectic flush, the scrofulous sores, and the pulmonary hemorrhages—gives these estimates a certain credibility. The standard history of tuberculosis is *The White Plague: Tuberculosis, Man and Society,* by René Dubos and Jean Dubos. For an analysis of the metaphoric significance of consumption during the nineteenth century, see Susan Sontag's "Illness as Metaphor."

3 Also known as the "pthisical aspect" and the "scrofulous diathesis," the "pthisical habitus" incorporated the totality of tubercular signs: emaciation, hectic fever, hacking cough, expectoration, hemorrhage, enlarged or abscessed glands, chest pain, painful joints, dyspepsia, and diarrhea. I am using the notion of the habitus more suggestively here, treating it as a sort of catchword for the peculiar sociology of consumption during this period. Pierre Bourdieu develops the concept of the habitus as a structure of existence in *Distinction: A Social Critique of the Judgement of Taste.*

4   In taking the notion of illness as metaphor for its subject matter, this study is deeply indebted to Susan Sontag's essays "Illness as Metaphor" and "AIDS and Its Metaphors," as well as to the growing body of work on the significance of illness to nineteenth-century thought. See Miriam Bailin, *The Sickroom in Victorian Fiction: The Art of Being Ill;* Sander Gilman, *Difference and Pathology: Stereotypes of Sexuality, Race, and Madness* and *Disease and Representation: Images of Illness from Madness to AIDS;* Bruce Haley, *The Healthy Body and Victorian Culture;* and Athena Vrettos, *Somatic Fictions: Imagining Illness in Victorian Culture.*

5   In relating disease to the broad cultural shifts entailed by industrial capitalism, I seek to contribute to the work of such critics as Nancy Armstrong, Catherine Gallagher, Mary Poovey, Anson Rabinbach, Elaine Scarry, Mark Seltzer, and Peter Stallybrass and Allon White on the politics of embodiment in machine culture. See Armstrong's *Desire and Domestic Fiction: A Political History of the Novel;* Gallagher's "The Bio-Economics of *Our Mutual Friend*" and "The Body versus the Social Body in the Works of Thomas Malthus and Henry Mayhew"; Poovey's *Making a Social Body: British Cultural Formation, 1830–1864;* Rabinbach's *The Human Motor: Energy, Fatigue, and the Origins of Modernity;* Scarry's *The Body in Pain: The Making and Unmaking of the World;* Seltzer's *Bodies and Machines;* and Stallybrass and White's *The Politics and Poetics of Transgression.*

6   See Gallagher's "The Bio-Economics of *Our Mutual Friend*" for a discussion of the Victorian tendency to couple questions of bodily and economic well-being in her essay.

7   At the beginning of the nineteenth century, only about 20 percent of the population of England and Wales lived in towns with more than five thousand inhabitants. Fifty years later more than half of the population was urban, and nearly 80 percent lived in cities by 1911. In 1801, London was the only city with a population above 100,000. Fifty years later there were ten cities of that size, and they were home to about 25 percent of the nation's population. By 1911 there were thirty-six such cities, and more than 40 percent of the population lived in them (Wohl 3).

8   The nineteenth century saw the birth of modern medicine. The standardization of medical education and the rise of the teaching hospital made the profession at once more respectable and more scientific. In addition to the advancements mentioned above, nineteenth-century medicine saw the rise of bacteriology and immunology; the refinement of surgery; the invention of the stethoscope, the kymograph, and the X ray; the articulation of cell theory and germ theory; the microscopic isolation of tuberculosis, cholera, anthrax, rabies, typhoid, and diphtheria; the birth of the pharmaceutical industry; the professionalization of modern nursing; and the entry of women into the medical profession. See W. F. Bynum's *Science and the Practice of Medicine in the Nineteenth Century* for an account of these events. The rise of the public health movement was inaugurated by James Phillips Kay's 1832 study of cholera in Manchester, and consolidated by Edwin Chadwick's *Report on the Sanitary Condition of the Labouring Population of Great Britain* in 1842. In 1846,

legislation regulating waste removal, public nuisances, and drainage systems began to be passed; the Public Health Act of 1848 marked the official entry of government into the regulation of public health. The act created a General Board of Health and empowered local authorities to establish systems for regulating everything from sewers, drains, water supplies, and waste removal to housing, burial grounds, parks, and public baths (Wohl 149). For an account of the rise of the public health movement in Victorian Britain, see Anthony S. Wohl, *Endangered Lives: Public Health in Victorian Britain.*

9   In 1843, the *Lancet,* a leading medical journal, published a table dramatizing comparative life expectancies across classes. In Bath, professionals and gentry could expect to live to fifty-five, farmers and tradesmen to thirty-seven, and laborers and artisans to twenty-five. The numbers were similar in Leeds (forty-four, twenty-seven, and nineteen, respectively), Bethnal Green (forty-five, twenty-six, and sixteen), Manchester (thirty-eight, twenty, and seventeen), and Liverpool (thirty-five, twenty-two, and fifteen) (quoted in Wohl 5).

10   The notion of occupational disease dates back to the ancient Egyptians. References to the injurious effects of work on health, and the occasional full-length study on occupational disease, appear periodically in Western literature from the fifteenth century on. The publication of Bernardino Ramazzini's *De Morbus Artificum Diatriba* (Diseases of workers) in 1713 marked the birth of the modern discourse on the subject. Ramazzini's work set the standards for both clinical practice and social critique, insisting that doctors could not diagnose patients without knowledge of their occupations, and providing the first fully systematic survey of the working conditions of different trades. Thackrah's treatise follows this basic paradigm and, with its original emphasis on the hazards of factory labor and machine work, set the tone for nineteenth-century treatments of the subject. Victorian writing about industrial disease culminated in two encyclopedic compendia: J. T. Arlidge's *The Hygiene Diseases and Mortality of Occupations* (1892) and Thomas Oliver's *Diseases of Occupation from the Legislative, Social, and Medical Points of View* (1908). For a brief survey of the history of writing about industrial disease, see Saul Benison's preface to Thackrah. For an account of Victorian attitudes toward industrial diseases, see Wohl's chapter "The Canker of Industrial Diseases."

11   White phosphorus, and not red, was responsible for matchmaker's necrosis. While phosphorus could be absorbed through the lungs and the skin, it was most often transferred from hand to mouth during match production. The consequence was a condition in which the lower face gradually rotted and fell away. On matchmaker's necrosis, see Arlidge 456–58, and Wohl 266–70. Wohl notes that the Salvation Army, in its efforts to publicize the unacceptable working conditions in shops and factories, took reporters and MPs to the homes of domestic matchmakers and then turned out the lights to dramatize the spectral effects of phosphorus on the flesh.

12   See Lombroso's *L'uomo delinquente* (1896), Geoffroy Saint-Hilaire and Cuvier's

Histoire naturelle des mammifères avec des figures originales (1824), and Tarnowsky's *Étude anthropométrique sur les prostituées et les voleuses* (1889). For an analysis of how iconographies of black female sexuality and the prostitute converged during the century, see Sander Gilman, "Black Bodies, White Bodies: Toward an Iconography of Female Sexuality in Late Nineteenth-Century Art, Medicine, and Literature."

13   Recent work on the Victorian body both charts the course of this ideological pattern and marks the fissures within it, the moments at which the totalizing framework of Victorian essentialism buckled under the pressure of its own over-determined determinism. The work on this subject is vast. For a representative sampling, see Gillian Beer, *Darwin's Plots: Evolutionary Narrative in Darwin, George Eliot, and Nineteenth-Century Fiction;* Sander Gilman, *Seeing the Insane* and "Black Bodies, White Bodies"; Ludmilla Jordanova, *Sexual Visions: Images of Gender in Science and Medicine between the Eighteenth and Twentieth Centuries;* Thomas Laqueur, *Making Sex: Body and Gender from the Greeks to Freud;* Anita Levy, *Other Women: The Writing of Class, Race, and Gender, 1832–1898;* Mary Poovey, "Scenes of an Indelicate Character: The Medical Treatment of Victorian Women"; Cynthia Eagle Russett, *Sexual Science: The Victorian Construction of Womanhood;* Elaine Showalter, *The Female Malady: Women, Madness, and Culture in England, 1830–1980;* and Sally Shuttleworth, "Female Circulation: Medical Discourse and Popular Advertising in the Mid-Victorian Era."

14   See in particular the chapters on commodity fetishism, the working day, and machinery and large-scale industry.

15   The full list of prices is reprinted in T. S. Crawford, *A History of the Umbrella* 191. Crawford's book records umbrellobilia from the ancient Egyptians to the present day. For more on Victorian umbrellas, see "Umbrellas in the East"; "Umbrellas"; and Robert Louis Stevenson, "The Philosophy of Umbrellas." On the many meaningful umbrellas in Dickens, see Edward T. Ward, "Gamps."

16   See Charles Dickens and Mark Lemon, "A Paper-Mill." For representative examples of vulcanization as a form of cultural assimilation, see T. O'Conor Sloane, *Rubber Hand Stamps and the Manipulation of India Rubber;* and B. F. Goodrich, *A Wonder Book of Rubber.* Goodrich writes that vulcanization "overcame the natural traits of rubber" by making it "dependable" (5), while Sloane writes that vulcanization resulted in a "healthy cure" of traits such as "susceptibility" (72, 14). This rhetoric of emotional management is refracted through an imperialist narrative of acquisition and acculturation: manufacturing treatises typically include detailed accounts of how rubber was collected by African, South American, and Indian natives; imported; "purified"; and then sold for use in industry and the home. For a modern history of rubber, see William Woodruff, *The Rise of the British Rubber Industry during the Nineteenth Century.*

I. ASIATIC CHOLERA AND THE RAW MATERIAL OF RACE

1 Although Nelson was Canadian, his attitude represents that of the major industrial nations of the West. England, France, Germany, and America all regarded cholera as an exotic scourge that posed a direct challenge to science and technology, and so threatened ideologies of progress. This attitude took on nationally specific forms in each country. This chapter concentrates on how cholera became a figure for distinctly English anxieties about the effect of industrialism on national identity.

2 Although cholera continued to plague Europe throughout the century, English public health reform, especially that centered on improved sewerage, the purification of the water supply, and the removal of "nuisances," had effectively eradicated cholera by 1866. English sanitation was never optimal—other contagious diseases continued to ravage the population throughout the century—but it eventually became good enough to keep out cholera. By 1896 cholera could be officially dismissed as a strictly "exotic disease." On cholera's role in the Victorian public health movement, see Wohl 118–25. On the history of Asiatic cholera in England, see Michael Durey, *The Return of the Plague: British Society and the Cholera 1831–2*; Norman Longmate, *King Cholera: The Biography of a Disease*; R. J. Morris, *Cholera, 1832: The Social Response to an Epidemic*; and Margaret Pelling, *Cholera, Fever and English Medicine, 1825–1865*. On cholera in America, see Charles Rosenberg, *The Cholera Years: The United States in 1832, 1849, and 1866*. On cholera in France, see François Delaporte, *Disease and Civilization: The Cholera in Paris, 1832*; for Germany, see Richard J. Evans, *Death in Hamburg: Society and Politics in the Cholera Years, 1830–1910*.

3 Asiatic cholera should not be confused with cholera nostras, a much milder form of intestinal disease common in the British Isles at that time. Like Asiatic cholera, cholera nostras was characterized by diarrhea, but it was significantly less virulent and was not considered contagious. Most people suffered from some form of enteritis during the summer months, when heat and damp fostered the growth of bacteria, which corrupted drinking water and caused food to spoil quickly. The difference between the two forms of cholera was dramatic, and in most cases there was no doubt about which was which. Cholera nostras was a minor endemic annoyance; cholera morbus (another name for the Asiatic variety) was a deadly modern plague. When Victorians wrote about "cholera," they invariably meant the Asiatic kind.

4 For a discussion of the French iconography of cholera, see Patrice Bourdelais and André Dodin, *Visages du Cholera*. The giant is from *La Caricature* (1831), the vagabond—embracing the July Revolution—is from a French broadside (1832), the corpse is from *Puck* (1883), the miasmatic cholera is from *Le Hanneton* (1867), the microbial cholera and the skeleton hosting dinner are from *Le Grelot* (1884), and the toreador is from *Le Courier Français* (1890). All of these are reprinted in

Bourdelais and Dodin, along with the portrait of cholera pumping water for the poor (no citation given).

5 "Fever" was a favorite diagnosis in the era before bacteriology made it possible to isolate pathogens. It encompassed everything from malaria to typhus to scarlet fever to a range of nonspecific agues, inflammations, and indispositions. On fever, see Margaret Pelling, *Cholera, Fever and English Medicine, 1825–1865;* and Wohl, *Endangered Lives.*

6 The inconsistency of Victorian images of exotic squalor, which were alternately African and Asiatic, is a characteristic gesture of what Edward Said has termed Orientalism, an ontology that consolidates imperial power by strategically failing to register differences within the category of the Other even as it insists on absolute distinctions between the Other and the Self, colonized and colonizer.

7 The logic of comparison that equated India with filth identified Calcutta in particular with the conditions that nurtured cholera. As one medical treatise expressed it, "Cholera is always present in Calcutta . . . one of the filthiest cities in the world. There is not a month in the year in which deaths do not occur from it, both European and native. It is the cause of one third of the total deaths, which vary from eleven thousand to sixteen thousand per year, out of a native population of about four hundred thousand" (Peters 21).

8 Brian Gardner's *The East India Company: A History* provides a detailed account of the incident in Calcutta; see pp. 75–80. Charles Dickens wrote two impassioned articles for the *Examiner* about the Tooting affair, using it as a vehicle for critiquing both the inhumane conditions at the school and the civic irresponsibility that enabled the school to exist: "The cholera broke out in Mr. Drouet's farm for children because it was brutally conducted, vilely kept, preposterously inspected, dishonestly defended, a disgrace to a Christian community, and a stain upon a civilised land" (quoted in Longmate 167). This diatribe is reminiscent of the one he had used a decade earlier to describe Squeers's school for boys in *Nicholas Nickleby* (1838–39).

9 According to Charles Creighton's seminal *History of Epidemics in Britain,* "The Indian or Asiatic cholera, which first showed itself on British soil in one or more houses of the Quay of Sunderland in the month of October, 1831, was a 'new disease' in a more real sense than anything in this country since the sweating sickness of 1485" (2:793).

10 James P. Kay's pioneering investigation of the living conditions of slums, *The Moral and Physical Condition of the Working Classes Employed in the Cotton Manufacture in Manchester* (1832), was written in direct response to the 1832 cholera epidemic.

11 *Choleraphobia* was a popular term for the widespread communal panic caused by the disease. Anxieties about infected food were not so far-fetched—cholera could live for a short time on green vegetables and survived up to five days on meat, milk, and cheese; sixteen days on apples; and two weeks in water (Wohl 120). Mayhew

notes that the street sellers themselves did not suffer from the contagious panic: "It does not appear that the costermongers manifested any personal dread of the visitation of the cholera, or thought that their lives were imperiled: 'We weren't a bit afraid,' said one of them, 'and, perhaps, that was the reason so few costers died of the cholera. I knew them all in Lambeth, I think, and I knew only one died of it, and he drank hard. Poor Waxy! he was a good fellow enough, and was well known in the Cut" (1:57–58).

12   Kingsley also uses the contagious commodity as a mode of social critique in his novel *Alton Locke: Tailor and Poet*, where it critiques oppressive social relations and outmoded models of contagion.

13   Historically, understandings of plague balanced a belief in divine intervention—a notion that still had power during the nineteenth century—against the inescapable conclusion that epidemic spread was closely tied to global expansion and the establishment of overseas markets. Time and again, plague was brought to Europe from Africa (yellow fever), Asia (bubonic plague), and America (Spanish explorers imported syphilis in exchange for smallpox) along with exotic goods. On transoceanic exchanges of disease, see William H. McNeill, *Plagues and Peoples* 176–207.

14   So important were Indian raw materials to English manufacture that England ran a trade deficit with India throughout the century. On England's place in the world economy, see Eric Hobsbawm, *Industry and Empire: The Making of Modern English Society: 1750 to the Present Day* 110–27.

15   Cholera came to England during the shift from regulated mercantilism to a laissez-faire policy of free trade. The repeal of the Corn Laws in 1846 marked an important shift in English attitudes toward foreign competition and goods. As English markets and manufacturing capabilities became more secure, England became more open to an economic policy that would enable it to buy food and raw materials on the cheapest markets and sell its manufactures on the most expensive ones. Asiatic cholera was the first truly modern pandemic. The development of a system of worldwide communication—railways, steamships, and overland routes—helped Asiatic cholera to spread faster and farther than any disease had before. The link between cholera and trade was acknowledged on a number of levels, most visibly in the ongoing debate about quarantine. Advocates stressed the need to protect the national health by restricting international trade; opponents focused on the economic hardship that would arise from effectively closing down ports.

16   In *The Human Motor: Energy, Fatigue, and the Origins of Modernity*, Anson Rabinbach argues that during the Victorian period, fatigue became one of the defining categories of lived experience. Registering the draining effects of social change on the bodily economy even as it compelled the organism to conserve its remaining energy, fatigue was both "a pathology and a prophylaxis against the demands of modernity" (11). See also Janet Oppenheim, *"Shattered Nerves": Doctors, Patients, and Depression in Victorian England;* and Edward Shorter, *From Paralysis to Fatigue: A History of Psychosomatic Illness in the Modern Era.*

17   Like cholera, the Great Exhibition of the Works of Industry of all Nations was a turbulence of novelty. For contemporary reactions to the Exhibition, see C. H. Gibbs-Smith, *The Great Exhibition of 1851* 26–32.

18   In *Science and the Practice of Medicine in the Nineteenth Century*, W. F. Bynum echoes early constructions of cholera, noting that "its novelty made it more awful" (74).

19   See W. Hamish Fraser, *The Coming of the Mass Market, 1850–1914*. Generally, historians date the coming of the mass market at around 1850, and treat the Great Exhibition of 1851 as the inauguration of commodity culture *tout court*. On the rise of commodity culture and the place of the Great Exhibition in developing a lasting semiotics of spectacle and material display, see Thomas Richards, *The Commodity Culture of Victorian England: Advertising and Spectacle, 1851–1914*. This chapter charts the prehistory of this commercial moment, tracking how anxieties about production, circulation, and exchange figured into early models of Asiatic cholera.

20   Charles Rosenberg develops the notion of epidemic disease as a social vector in *The Cholera Years*. Rosenberg argues that a secular shift in American values can be charted through changing attitudes toward cholera between 1832 and 1866. In *Dangerous Sexualities: Medico-Moral Politics in England since 1830*, Frank Mort makes a similar argument about cholera as a vector of social mores, using it as an example of how Victorians tended to moralize disease by linking contagion to the spread of bad behavior. For a more wide-ranging theory of how epidemics have historically been narrated, see Rosenberg's *Explaining Epidemics and Other Studies in the History of Medicine*.

21   Before germ theory, models of contagion were hotly debated and the mechanism of epidemic spread was open to any number of inventive interpretations. While it was clear that cholera had followed the major European trade routes on its trip from India to England, no one knew precisely how the disease was transmitted. Contagionists believed that it was spread by contact with infected people, food, and things; supporters of zymotic, or miasmic, theory argued that cholera arose spontaneously from the squalor of slums, originating in and emanating from accumulated filth and decay. Simon's theory of disease as the result of atmospheric "poisons" was typical of early and mid-Victorian epidemiology. As Edwin Chadwick, a major advocate of miasmic theory, put it, "All smell is, if it be intense, immediate acute disease" (quoted in Bynum 72). Theories of spread universally combined ideas about miasma and moral vulnerability: the poor were sick more often, they argued, not only because there were more pathogenic sources of stench in the slums, but also because their filthy habits made them extremely liable to infection. Neither theory could account for cholera's erratic patterns, which could decimate some populations while sparing others, and could even strike one side of a street while leaving the other alone. Not until 1859, when John Snow and William Farr demonstrated a decisive link between the London water supply and patterns of spread, did cholera begin to be understood as a waterborne disease that

was communicated orally, either by drinking contaminated fluids or by inadvertent transmission of choleraic purgings to the mouth. The cholera bacillus was not isolated until 1884, when the German bacteriologist Robert Koch advanced the first fully satisfactory explanation of epidemic infection. By then, Asiatic cholera had been consolidated in a peculiar mixture of medical and metaphorical language, a scientific method of imagining in which symptoms and patterns of spread were used to describe a deeply symbolic account of cultural contamination and collapse. On Victorian theories of communicable disease, see Margaret Pelling, *Cholera, Fever and English Medicine, 1825–1865.*

22   Concerns over water purification were especially intense following the 1848–49 epidemic, and were heightened by the publication of A. H. Hassall's composite drawings of what lived in London water. Published in color plates in his 1850 *Microscopical Examination of the Water Supplied to the Inhabitants of London and Suburban Districts,* they were reprinted in the *Lancet* in 1851 and included in Hassall's 1876 opus on adulteration, *Food: Its Adulterations, and the Methods for Their Detection. Punch* did a send-up of Hassall's work in 1850, depicting a drop of London water as a crowded decoction of "aldermen, deputies, common councilmen . . . disporting in the liquid filth as in their native element" ("A Drop of London Water" 188). On the history of water purification, see Christopher Hamlin, *A Science of Impurity.*

23   It took very little cholera to contaminate the water supply. In 1866, the chemist Edward Frankland showed that an extremely dilute solution containing one part cholera evacuations to one thousand parts water was pure poison. On Frankland, see Hamlin, *Science of Impurity* 152–77.

24   The blackening caused by cholera was the combined effect of dehydration (which darkened the blood) and tissue necrosis. The characteristic cramping of cholera was due to dehydration. The contractile spasms of victims were dramatic—limbs could twitch for hours after death, and some corpses even sat up. The peculiarly animate morbidity of cholera patients fueled fears about premature burial that were especially intense during the cholera outbreak of 1832, when the Anatomy Act legalized the dissection of unclaimed pauper bodies. The spastic active corpses of cholera victims seemed to give substance to claims that doctors were declaring live bodies dead and then exhuming them for purposes of dissection. In *Death, Dissection and the Destitute,* Ruth Richardson outlines the intimate connections between the social histories of cholera and dissection; see pp. 223–29. On funeral customs and premature burial during the nineteenth century, see Martin Pernick, "Back from the Grave: Recurring Controversies over Defining and Diagnosing Death in History."

25   The article paraphrases John W. Draper's *Human Physiology* (1856).

26   A tendency to conflate the African and the ape was typical of nineteenth-century attitudes toward race. The coming of cholera coincided with the upsurge of interest in the origins of races, as evidenced by the founding of the Royal Geographical

Society in 1830, the Ethnological Society of London in 1843, and the Anthropological Society in 1863. Cholera coincided with the shift from Enlightenment linguistic models of racial difference to the emphasis on physical characteristics such as brain weight, facial characteristics, skin color, and body type that characterized Victorian theories of difference. On Victorian theories of race, see George Stocking, *Victorian Anthropology;* and Christine Bolt, *Victorian Attitudes to Race.*

27 Linking race and industry by refracting them through the lens of contagious disease, the discourse of cholera added a distinctly modern dimension to what was by the nineteenth century a long-standing association between blackness and disease in Western thought. See Sander Gilman, "On the Nexus of Blackness and Madness."

28 See Peter Keating, ed., *Into Unknown England 1866–1913: Selections from the Social Explorers,* for examples of how a rhetoric of primitivism modulated English social criticism.

29 Certain occupations were thought to confer a kind of elemental immunity to cholera, building up a resistance in workers by exposing them to the stuff that infection would turn them into. Metalworkers—particularly those dealing in copper and steel—and charcoal manufacturers were thought to be comparatively immune (Jameson 260; Tardieu 254), while coal miners were thought to be some of the most susceptible people since the mineshaft was, as John Snow remarked, their privy as well as their place of work.

30 The plot of *Poor Miss Finch* hinges on the central character's efforts to keep his darkened complexion a secret from his fiancée, whose blindness has produced in her a phobic horror of dark people and things. Racial overtones aside, Collins's portrayal of dermal darkening is actually scientifically accurate: in silver nitrate poisoning, molecules of silver really do oxidize in the skin, tarnishing it a deep dusky gray.

31 By midcentury, specially designed mechanical devices were replacing the small boys used to clean chimneys. Mayhew notes that "the 'brush,' technically called 'the head'" of the machine, is made of "elastic whalebone spikes, which 'give' and bend, in accordance with the up or down motion communicated by the man working the machine" (2:356). If the head of the sweep resembles his machine, the machine in turn approximates a human head.

32 See Sontag's "AIDS and Its Metaphors" for a reading of cholera's importance to nationalist discourses of the late nineteenth and early twentieth centuries.

33 I refer to the subtitle of Anderson's *Imagined Communities: Reflections on the Origin and Spread of Nationalism.*

34 Another instance of this semiotic spread: the examples cited here from During, Hutcheon, and Brydon are all collected in the recent *Post-Colonial Studies Reader* (ed. Ashcroft, Griffiths, and Tiffin), where their cross-contaminations are held up as an exemplary exchange of ideas.

35 Said's infectious rhetoric has been latent in his prose for years. An early instance

can be found in the introduction to *The World, the Text, and the Critic* (1983), which makes a case for "secular criticism" by pointing out the noxious sterility of then-contemporary literary theory, whose "peculiar mode of appropriating its subject matter . . . is *not* to appropriate anything that is worldly, circumstantial, or socially contaminated. 'Textuality' is the somewhat mystical and disinfected subject matter of literary theory" (3).

36 I am speaking here specifically of the symbolic dimensions of cholera. Medical historians have documented the role of cholera and other contagious diseases in the establishment and maintenance of colonial rule. These studies focus on material patterns of spread, issues of policy, and the practice of military and indigenous medicine. See David Arnold, *Colonizing the Body: State Medicine and Epidemic Disease in Nineteenth-Century India* and *Imperial Medicine and Indigenous Societies;* Anil Kumar, *Medicine and the Raj: British Medical Policy in India, 1835–1911;* and Roy M. MacLeod and Milton James Lewis, *Disease, Medicine and Empire: Perspectives on Western Medicine and the Experience of European Expansion.*

37 For a detailed analysis of Mann's depiction of Asiatic cholera, see Laura Otis, *Membranes: Metaphors of Invasion in Nineteenth-Century Literature, Science, and Politics.* Tracing links in German writing among cholera, creativity, and colonialism, Otis's chapter is a useful reminder of how widespread this symbolic conformation was.

38 In a headier vein, Anne McClintock writes in *Imperial Leather: Race, Gender, and Sexuality in the Colonial Contest* that "the disciplinary quarantine of psychoanalysis from history was germane to imperial modernity" (8).

2. BREAST REDUCTIONS

1 My etymology of *income* is based on the *OED*'s entry for that word.

2 "Rab and His Friends" was first published in Brown's *Horae Subsecivae* (1858), a collection of light anecdotes dedicated to showing the importance of humor and humanity in the care of the sick. It was reprinted in 1859 as a separate tale.

3 I use the term *political economy* broadly here to include not only critiques of the factory system by writers such as Carlyle, Marx, and Engels, but also attendant discourses of social analysis: reports on sanitary conditions by the likes of Chadwick and Kay; analyses of prostitution by men such as Acton, Greg, and Parent-Duchâtelet; the sociology of the urban poor produced by Mayhew and later Booth; and the nascent theories of mass culture articulated at the turn of the century by Gustave Le Bon and Gabriel Tarde. Nancy Armstrong and Anita Levy term the same discourse "sociology" in *Desire and Domestic Fiction* and *Other Women.* More recently, in *Making a Social Body,* Mary Poovey calls the language I am describing "anatomical realism." Clearly, there is a certain amount of ambiguity surrounding the proper generic designation of the vastly varied writing that grew up in response to industrialization during the nineteenth century. I prefer *political economy* to

sociology or *anatomical realism* because that term bears more relation to the Victorians' own generic categories than the more recent designations.

4 See L. J. Rather's *Genesis of Cancer: A Study in the History of Ideas* for a medical history of the disease. Rather is particularly informative about the impact of cell theory on concepts of cancer.

5 The standard history of breast cancer is Daniel de Moulin's *A Short History of Breast Cancer.* See also Carl M. Mansfield's *Early Breast Cancer: Its History and Results of Treatment.* I am less interested in recapitulating Victorian debates about causation, diagnosis, and treatment than in elucidating the imaginative structures that underlie the discourse as a whole.

6 Men could develop breast cancer, but it was extremely rare (Paget estimated that 2 percent of all cases were males [cited in Gross 238]) and was regarded largely as a feminine anomaly occurring in incompletely gendered men. As James Compton Burnett writes in *Tumours of the Breast, and Their Treatment and Cure by Medicines* (1888), "Of course men get tumours also, but that is by reason of their being the sons of women, and possessing some of their formative power thus perverted and locally expressed" (165). Samuel Gross surveys the literature on male breast cancer in his short chapter "Tumors of the Male Mammary Gland" 237–38. See also John Birkett, "Disease of the Gland in the Male," in *The Diseases of the Breast and Their Treatment* 253–58; and A. Marmaduke Sheild, "Diseases of the Male Breast," in *A Clinical Treatise on Diseases of the Breast* 482–98.

7 Historians agree that the breast became the privileged locus of femininity during the eighteenth century. Ludmilla Jordanova writes that "breasts not only symbolized the most fundamental social bond—that between mother and child—they were also the means by which families were made, since their beauty elicited the desires of the male for the female" (29). Ruth Perry details the significance of the breast to bourgeois notions of female sexuality in "Colonizing the Breast: Sexuality and Maternity in Eighteenth-Century England." See Londa Schiebinger's *Nature's Body: Gender in the Making of Modern Science* for an account of how the breast figured in the creation of the category "mammalia" during the eighteenth century. For a study of the historical significance of breasts from antiquity on, see Marilyn Yalom, *A History of the Breast.* For analyses of Victorian constructions of femininity as an essential, biologically based phenomenon, see Thomas Laqueur, *Making Sex;* and Cynthia Eagle Russett, *Sexual Science.*

8 See Engels, "Single Branches of Industry," in *The Condition of the Working Class in England* 144–96.

9 Where critiques of the manufacturing system posited a fundamental impasse between factories and families, and embodied this impasse in the figure of the enervated female worker, arguments in favor of mechanization sought to reconcile labor and femininity by arguing that factories brought out women's essential nature. See Nancy Armstrong's *Desire and Domestic Fiction* 169–76 for a discussion of the gender politics of reform literature.

10 The contemporary medical distinction between organic and functional disorders

was begun during the nineteenth century. Functional disorders were nervous diseases without an identifiable organic cause, such as a lesion or nerve injury. Hysteria, hypochondria, neurosis, and neurasthenia were all functional disorders.

11 Blushing, dimpling, and puckering were all signs of breast cancer, as were bossiness, indolence, and tension. For representative examples, see Sheild 344, 358, 369; Burnett 138; and Deaver and McFarland 533. Dimpling in particular was a clear indicator of cancer: "In a large proportion of the cases, the skin is obviously dimpled, and there is no sign of more vital import than this. The slightest dimple on the skin of the mamma of an elderly woman, is a dangerous symptom which cannot be ignored or neglected by any medical man" (Sheild 345). In inflamed cancer, or "brawny cancer," "the skin has a peculiar roseate erythematous blush upon it (cancer erythema), which spreads over the skin of the mamma and thorax, gradually fading off into the surrounding tissues. There is local heat and tenderness, and the bodily temperature is raised" (Sheild 358). The technical term for hard cancer was "schirrous," which meant "rock." The pathological progression of cancer was commonly referred to as the "degeneration" of tissues; James Paget called cancer a "disease of degeneracy" (cited in Nunn 180). On irritation as an exciting cause of cancer, see Deaver and McFarland 337. As these examples show, the Victorian and early-twentieth-century vocabulary of cancer draws heavily on the language of sensibility, a deeply gendered discourse of feeling. For a discussion of the gendering of sensibility at the end of the eighteenth century, see John Mullan, *Sentiment and Sociability: The Language of Feeling in the Eighteenth Century*. On Victorian sensibility, see Karen Halttunen, *Confidence Men and Painted Women: A Study of Middle-Class Culture in America, 1830–1870*.

12 Body parts that spontaneously mimicked diseases were not unusual. James Paget lectured on the phenomenon, which he called "nervous mimicry" or "neuromimesis," noting that the breast was particularly liable to nervous delusion in the form of "phantom tumours," painful masses that weren't actually there. See Paget, "Nervous Mimicry (Neuromimesis) of Tumors," in *Clinical Lectures and Essays* 233–51. For more on phantom tumors of the breast, see Mitchell, *Lectures on Diseases of the Nervous System, Especially in Women* 107–8; and Sheild, "Phantom Tumours" 372–75. Mitchell very nearly sent one of his patients to surgery to have her extremely realistic phantom tumor removed.

13 For ease of reference I have cited single page numbers from a small selection of authors here. They are meant, however, as simple index points. References to eggs, nuts, cheeses, and so on are everywhere in Victorian descriptions of tumors.

14 Depending on its origins, cancer could take a variety of forms. The basic categories were schirrous, encephaloid, melanoid (rare), fibroplastic or colloid, epithelial (rare), and keloid (rare). Schirrous, which some physicians considered to be the only "true" cancer, was hard and poorly circumscribed, growing in rough, irregular tumors or in plates. It tended to alter the "character" of the breast by "hardening" it rather than deforming it (Velpeau 348). Patients often described schirrous cancer as an "iron-like cage" encircling and stifling them (Velpeau 343, 345). Atrophic

schirrous, a subset of schirrous proper, shriveled organs and tissues, retracting the nipple and eating away the breast's flesh. Encephaloid, or medullary, cancer presents as a round lump, movable but not wholly independent of the surrounding tissues. Lardaceous tumors are firm, and as they grow they form a shiny, discolored "boss" on the surface of the breast; fungous or knotted encephaloid tumors are lobulated, "soft, elastic, and supple" (361), tending toward the surface of the breast rather than its base. These are the fastest-growing, largest forms of cancer. Fibroplastic tumors are generally hard and compact; they are slow growing and deep and can soften into spongy, gelatinous material over time. See Velpeau 335–86.

15   Mayhew's *London Labour and the London Poor* (1861) provides an elaborate compendium of the goods sold on London streets at midcentury. There is an uncanny overlap between the edibles hawked on London streets and those that appear in cancerous breasts. On the street sale of butter, cheese, and eggs, see vol. 1:135; for oranges, apples, and nuts, see 1:90–94.

16   On buttery and cheesy tumors, see Velpeau, "Butter-like Tumours" 56–59.

17   See, for example, *The Eighteenth Brumaire of Louis Bonaparte* 267.

18   I discuss Virchow's comparison of organism to state in detail later in this chapter.

19   *Combination* referred to any union or organization of workers; combinations were associated with conspiracy, the threat of violence, and even revolution. Illegal at the turn of the century, unions had gained a certain amount of respectability by the 1850s. See E. P. Thompson, *The Making of the English Working Class* 500–516.

20   On crowd theory, see Jaap van Ginneken, *Crowds, Psychology, and Politics: 1871–1899;* and Robert Nye, *The Origins of Crowd Psychology: Gustave Le Bon and the Crisis of Mass Democracy in the Third Republic.*

21   The notion of the breast as a bad neighborhood goes both ways: Jacob Riis calls the tenement and the saloon the "twin breasts" that nourish poverty in his 1890 analysis of New York's Lower East Side, *How the Other Half Lives: Studies among the Tenements of New York.*

22   Creighton develops the notion of cancer as a buildup of waste throughout his study. See his chapter "The Lymphatic Glands of the Breast in Connexion with the Disposal of Its Cellular Waste" 57–82, and "Tumours Formed by Waste Cells of the Nuclear Kind" (*Contributions* 121–48). On duct cancer, see Sheild 314–20.

23   James Paget notes the breast's vulnerability to rodent ulcers in his description of malignant papillary dermatitis (otherwise known as Paget's disease of the nipple) (reprinted in Sheild 686–87, with picture).

24   Breast cancer discourse framed masses as miniature crowds well before Le Bon developed his theory in his *Psychologie des foules* (1895). My point is not to suggest that medicine is quoting these formulations, or even actively referring to them. I mean to be far more suggestive here and want simply to note how much conceptual energy is shared by the seemingly unrelated discourses of breast cancer and social theory. Indeed, the ultimate aim of this analysis is to pose precisely the problem of their relation. The second half of this chapter deals specifically with the historical and methodological dimensions of this question.

25 See William Acton, *Prostitution;* W. R. Greg, "Prostitution"; and Bracebridge Hemyng, "Prostitution in London" for fine examples of Victorian writing about prostitution. See also Amanda Anderson, *Tainted Souls and Painted Faces: The Rhetoric of Fallenness in Victorian Culture;* and Judith Walkowitz, *Prostitution and Victorian Society: Women, Class, and the State.*

26 *Extirpation* was a standard medical term for the removal of cancerous tissue. It was used as a synonym for amputation, and was also used to indicate the comparatively minor operation known today as lumpectomy. *Mastectomy* did not become the term for the removal of the breast until the twentieth century.

27 For a discussion of how metonymic slippages between body and slum character-ized Victorian conceptions of the city, see Stallybrass and White, *The Politics and Poetics of Transgression,* "The City: The Sewer, the Gaze, the Contaminating Touch."

28 Separate-sphere ideology constructed women as essentially private and domestic. The constitutive elements of public space were seen as threatening to the values that women embodied, even as they made those values visible (by contrast) and inevitably participated in their construction: the domestic woman was a judicious consumer of commodities; the crowd was a feminine, feminizing entity; and the slum was morally tainted in large part because poor women necessarily led such public lives. On women as consumers, see Nancy Armstrong, "The Rise of the Domestic Woman," in *Desire and Domestic Fiction* 59–95; and Thomas Richards, "Those Lovely Seaside Girls," in *The Commodity Culture of Victorian England* 205–48. On the femininity of crowds, see Gustave Le Bon, "The Sentiments and Morality of Crowds," in *The Crowd* 15–44; on the slum as the scene of female corruption, see Anita Levy, "Sociology: Disorder in the House of the Poor," in *Other Women* 20–47; and Stallybrass and White, *The Politics and Poetics of Trans-gression,* "The City: The Sewer, the Gaze, and the Contaminating Touch" 125–48.

29 For a critique of the synecdochal reasoning that enables much "cultural studies" work, see Michael Schudson's "Paper Tigers." Carolyn Porter addresses this issue in her critique of the new historicism's current fascination with the "riveting anec-dote" ("History and Literature: 'After the New Historicism'" 261). According to Porter, by turning the anecdote into a "synecdoche . . . for a larger cultural pattern which it simultaneously invokes and provides the only evidence for," we have installed a "colonialist formalism" in the name of radical history ("Are We Being Historical Yet?" 778–79). See also Mark Seltzer's observations about cultural stud-ies's tendency to flatten connections into equivalencies by relying too heavily on analogies. Seltzer's concept of "cultural logistics" issues an important corrective: "Things are in part what they appear to be and . . . nothing is simply reducible to anything else" ("Serial Killers (1)" 120).

30 The list of foundational feminist-Victorianist work in both literary and cultural history goes on and on. Other important titles include Nina Auerbach, *Commu-nities of Women: An Idea in Fiction* (1978) and *Woman and the Demon: The Life of a Victorian Myth* (1982); Sandra Gilbert and Susan Gubar, *The Madwoman in the*

Attic: The Woman Writer and the Nineteenth-Century Literary Imagination (1979); Elaine Showalter, *A Literature of Their Own: British Women Novelists from Brontë to Lessing* (1976); and Carroll Smith-Rosenberg, *Disorderly Conduct: Visions of Gender in Victorian America* (1985).

31   See Michel Foucault's *History of Sexuality*, vol. 1, which grounds its discursive theory of sex in a cursory account of Victorian repression. I read Foucault's "history" less as a lesson in nineteenth-century cultural formation than as a lesson in how the idea of nineteenth-century culture can provide a proving ground for contemporary theory.

32   See Scott's chapter "Gender: A Useful Category of Historical Analysis," in *Gender and the Politics of History;* and Sedgwick's "Axiomatic," in *Epistemology of the Closet.*

33   On the recuperation of the hysteric as a figure for revolt, see Hélène Cixous and Catherine Clément, *The Newly Born Woman* 271–96; and Dianne Hunter, "Hysteria, Psychoanalysis, and Feminism: The Case of Anna O." On anorexia as a synecdochal sign of various social pathologies, see Susan Bordo, "Anorexia Nervosa: Psychopathology as the Crystallization of Culture," in *Unbearable Weight: Feminism, Western Culture, and the Body;* Gillian Brown, "Anorexia, Humanism, and Feminism"; Susie Orbach, *Hunger Strike: The Anorectic's Struggle as a Metaphor for Our Age;* and Naomi Wolf, *The Beauty Myth: How Images of Beauty Are Used against Women.*

34   Christina Crosby makes a related argument in her essay "Reading the Victorians," which notes the tendency of feminist work on nineteenth-century gender ideology to get "caught in a kind of mirror relation" to its subject matter. For a more general critique of gender as a potentially tautological category of analysis, see Mark Bauerlein, *Literary Criticism: An Autopsy.*

35   My thinking here is indebted to Diana Fuss's account of how constructivist feminisms are predicated on essentialist logic. See *Essentially Speaking: Feminism, Nature and Difference.*

36   Christina Crosby calls for such a self-consciously literary approach to history writing in "Reading the Victorians," noting that in the wake of Foucault, Victorian studies has become peculiarly telegraphic, especially when it comes to gender analysis. For a more general treatment of the question of criticism's implication in its construction of the past, see David Simpson's collection, *Subject to History: Ideology, Class, Gender.* For a variety of perspectives on the place of the "literary"— read close reading—in cultural studies, see the March 1997 Forum in *PMLA.* For a useful summary of historians' own mixed response to the so-called linguistic turn of certain radical branches of historiography, see Christopher Kent's review essay, "Victorian Social History: Post-Thompson, Post-Foucault, Postmodern." Kent's essay is particularly valuable for its explanation of what Foucault and the interdisciplinary movement he has inspired have meant for the discipline of history.

37   I owe much here to Mary Poovey's *Making a Social Body: British Cultural Formation, 1830–1864.* Poovey's book conducts an ongoing interrogation of totalizing historical frameworks—insisting on close reading as the mainstay of responsible

historical practice and noting too the connections between Victorian conceptions of gender and certain epistemological schisms in contemporary feminism. As such, it stands not simply as a revisionist history of the body's place in British cultural formation, but also as an attempt to revise our models for thinking history itself.

38 On the rise of cell theory with particular emphasis on its relation to cancerology, see Rather's chapters "Cell Theory and the Genesis of Cells in Tumors, 1838–52" and "Cell Theory and the Genesis of Cells in Tumors, 1852–1900," in *Genesis of Cancer*. On Virchow's place in modern cell theory, see Rather's essays "The Place of Virchow's *Cellular Pathology* in Medical Thought" and "Harvey, Virchow, Bernard, and the Methodology of Science." Virchow's *Cellular Pathology* (1858) is considered to be the single most important medical treatise of the nineteenth century. It was translated into English in 1860.

39 Virchow's attack is directed specifically at German thinkers, who, he felt, were importing the Hegelian dialectic into a field where it did not belong; but it may be generalized to medicine at large.

40 For a discussion of Virchow's opinion of scientific method as it was practiced during the late eighteenth and early nineteenth centuries, see Rather, "Harvey, Virchow, Bernard, and the Methodology of Science."

41 This is implicitly an argument with the popular methodological concept of cultural poetics, by which we have come to describe the project of bringing "the literary," or close textual analysis, to cultural critique. Derived from the Geertzian notion of "interpretive anthropology," cultural poetics is most firmly associated with 1980s new historicism, especially the work of Stephen Greenblatt. It became the guiding ethos of American cultural studies in the 1990s, so much so that it is no longer necessary to invoke or even reference the term. "Resonance" is a principal concept in cultural poetics, whose basic premise is one of essential connectedness. As Greenblatt puts it, the term speaks to "the power of the object displayed to reach out beyond its formal boundaries to a larger world, to evoke in the viewer the complex, dynamic cultural forces from which it has emerged and for which as metaphor or more simply as metonymy it may be taken by a viewer to stand" (170). A number of critics have articulated objections to such a methodological premise. Mark Bauerlein sees it as a self-serving analytical construct that enables critics to hedge their interdisciplinary bets: "Cultural poetics is cultural, but not quite historical, aesthetic, but not quite formalist. To represent culture, it draws analogies whose justification is epistemological, not logical or historical. . . . The analogies may have little basis in fact and form, but so long as they bring about the defamiliarizing cognition, they count as legitimate instances of cultural poetics inquiry" (26). Carolyn Steedman and Carolyn Porter have also written persuasively on this subject. In her essays "History and Literature" and "Are We Being Historical Yet?" Porter argues that all too often, the importation of close reading into historical work does less to make new kinds of knowledge available than it does to reinscribe a limiting and ultimately misleading formalism based on what she

calls—after Walter Cohen—"a principle of arbitrary connectedness" ("History and Literature" 261). Steedman's "Culture, Cultural Studies, and the Historians" cites Porter and Dominick La Capra in her characterization of how the "trance-like reliance on culture as a principle of connection and coherence" has blinded us to "transformation" because it ensures that we can see only what it tells us to see: "the connectedness of everything" (616). This chapter is in part an attempt to assess the costs of such a premise and an effort to imagine what history would look like if we continued to hear resonances but refused to yoke them together in a causal or totalizing analytical framework. In this sense, it draws inspiration from Lawrence Grossberg's concept of articulation, the term he uses to describe the necessary but inevitably oxymoronic project of a properly judicious cultural studies: to describe the "relations of a non-relation" ("Toward a Genealogy of the State of Cultural Studies" 144).

42   See Mary Poovey's "The Production of Abstract Space," in *Making a Social Body*, for an elaboration of this concept.

43   For an excellent overview of feminism's relation to science, see Evelyn Fox Keller and Helen E. Longino, eds., *Feminism & Science*. The collection provides a clear history of the feminist critique of science since the 1970s and reprints a fine selection of major work in the field. See especially the essays by Keller, Emily Martin, Londa Schiebinger, and Nancy Leys Stepan on scientific metaphor.

44   The difficulty of reconciling a strong sentimental attachment to the breast with a necessary clinical detachment was a direct result of eighteenth-century conceptions of breast cancer, which routinely depicted the diseased breast as a problem of gender. This association manifested itself differently in different spaces. In Maria Edgeworth's *Belinda* (1801), Lady Delacour's diseased breast not only reflects her poor mothering and penchant for dueling, but spontaneously cures itself—on the eve of her mastectomy, no less—when she repents and reforms. Operations that preserved the appearance of the breast—especially the nipple—were favored surgical techniques. Fanny Burney's harrowing account of her 1812 mastectomy reads much like a patient's view of Warren's later tale, with its descriptions of tearful, blood-spattered surgeons and its touching portrait of Burney's overwhelming desire to protect her fragile husband from worry. For Victorian physicians, the emotional burden of mastectomy had as much to do with the previous century's symbolic legacy as it did with the poor prognosis of cancer patients. On breast cancer in eighteenth-century literature and culture, see Ruth Perry's *The Celebrated Mary Astell: An Early English Feminist*. On eighteenth-century surgeries for breast cancer, see D'Arcy Power, "The History of the Amputation of the Breast to 1904." On Burney's mastectomy letter, see Julia Epstein, *The Iron Pen: Frances Burney and the Politics of Women's Writing*.

45   As so often happens with scientific breakthroughs, Halsted's work was paralleled by that of a colleague, Willy Meyer. Meyer published his own report on radical mastectomy shortly after Halsted presented his findings. On the history of mastectomy, see D'Arcy Power, "The History of the Amputation of the Breast

to 1904"; and William Cooper, "The History of the Radical Mastectomy." The major writings on breast cancer from the ancients on, including more than a dozen nineteenth-century articles and reports, are reprinted in Guy Robbins's *Silvergirl's Surgery: The Breast*. Daniel de Moulin's *Short History of Breast Cancer* provides a useful table of statistics regarding mastectomy survival rates.

46 Of course, radical mastectomy has not been quite the boon that Halsted, Meyer, and others predicted it would be. It has recently come under fire as an unnecessarily extreme technique, and more and more women are now treated with comparatively minor surgeries that leave the affected breast relatively intact. And, of course, the notion of a cure for breast cancer that involves neither radiation nor chemotherapy sounds utterly naive to us today. Nonetheless, the 1890s marked a profound revolution in the management of breast cancer, one whose psychological impact was at least as important as its practical innovations (breast cancer cannot, after all, be cured unless we believe that it can be).

47 Here I depart from the feminist reading of the history of mastectomy, which sees Victorian medicine's treatment of the female body as fraught with an oppressive sexual politics. While I do not dispute that women's bodies are objectified in medical accounts of mastectomy, I do take issue with an analytical stance that neither acknowledges the tactical nature of that objectification (preferring instead to see it as a sign of an unenlightened misogyny) nor appreciates the very real material benefits of that strategic objectification: saving women's lives. Certainly misogynistic attitudes toward women filter through the literature on breast cancer, as they do through much of the medical writing during the period. But it is reductive to read that literature as an allegory of oppression. For different viewpoints on the sexual politics of mastectomy during this period, see Judith Fryer, "'The Body in Pain' in Thomas Eakins' *Agnew Clinic*"; and Mary Jacobus, "Baring the Breast: Mastectomy and the Surgical Analogy."

48 For fine examples of each, see Emily Martin, "The Egg and the Sperm: How Science has Constructed a Romance Based on Stereotypical Male-Female Roles"; and Nancy Leys Stepan, "Race and Gender: The Role of Analogy in Science."

3. FRACTIONS OF MEN: ENGENDERING AMPUTATION

1 Mitchell was one of the most important figures in nineteenth-century medicine. Specializing in the new science of neurology, he wrote definitive studies on nerve injuries—particularly those suffered by Civil War soldiers, on the nervous diseases of women, and on related problems of energy and fatigue. He was also a prolific novelist and short story writer. Mitchell's work on nerve injury and neurasthenia was well known and much respected: British physicians regularly prescribed Mitchell's famous rest cure in cases of extreme nervous distress, and his theories were so influential that they made their way beyond the clinical context into contemporary materialist philosophy. In *Problems of Life and Mind* (1879–80) for example, the English intellectual George Henry Lewes uses Mitchell's work on

amputation to develop his portrait of the mind-body relationship: "The phantom limb of which Weir Mitchell speaks, is only one detail in the general picture mentally formed of the body" (336). More than any other figure, Mitchell set the tone for Victorian attitudes toward amputation. His popular stories and medical studies established the terms through which amputation—as a pathology and as a philosophical problem—would be apprehended in both Britain and America for the rest of the century. On Mitchell, see Drinka 197–209. For a related reading of Mitchell's "Case of George Dedlow," see Walter Benn Michaels, *The Gold Standard and the Logic of Naturalism: American Literature at the Turn of the Century* 23–25.

2   Many books attempting to articulate the relationship between mind and body were published during the nineteenth century. Alexander Bain, like Maudsley, posited an absolute interdependence of the two, writing in *Mind and Body: The Theories of Their Relation* (1873) that because "the mind is completely at the mercy of the bodily condition . . . [b]odily affliction is often the cause of a total change in the moral nature" (41, 9). Mitchell's story draws on the rigid somaticism of such materialist medicine, although it is worth noting that there were some significant dissenting voices. Sir Benjamin Brodie, for instance, argues in *Mind and Matter; or, Physiological Inquiries* (1857) that while the "connexion between the mind and body is in many instances too palpable to be overlooked," it is yet "wholly inconceivable that any exaltation of the known properties of matter should produce the conscious indivisible monad which [a man feels himself] to be" (232, 36).

3   Men wounded in the Civil and Crimean Wars made up the majority of amputees, although it was estimated that the annual rate of amputations due to industrial accidents rivaled that of wartime. As *Scientific American* wrote in 1895, although "our war has long passed . . . the electric motor and steam engine continue to make as many cripples as did the missiles of war" ("Improved Artificial Limbs" 52).

4   Bruce Haley elegantly draws out the importance of wholeness to Victorian concepts of health, particularly to men's health, in *The Healthy Body and Victorian Culture*. On Victorian manliness as a function of physical culture, see J. A. Mangan and James Walvin's *Manliness and Morality: Middle-Class Masculinity in Britain and America, 1800–1940*, especially the chapters on muscular Christianity, athletics, and boys' schools.

5   On the Great Exhibition as the originary moment of modern consumer culture, see Thomas Richards, "The Great Exhibition of Things," in *The Commodity Culture of Victorian England*. On World War I's impact on mutilation, see Seth Koven, "Remembering and Dismemberment: Crippled Children, Wounded Soldiers, and the Great War in Great Britain"; and Joanna Bourke, *Dismembering the Male: Men's Bodies, Britain and the Great War*.

6   There is a small but remarkably good body of work on the significance of amputation and prosthesis in the specific national contexts of Britain and America between 1850 and World War I. On the British meanings of mutilation, see Bourke, Koven, and Albert Hutter, "Dismemberment and Articulation in *Our Mutual Friend*." On mutilation in an American context, see Laurann Figg and Jane Farrell

Beck, "Amputation in the Civil War: Physical and Social Dimensions"; Leslie Katz, "Flesh of His Flesh: Amputation in *Moby Dick* and S. W. Mitchell's Medical Papers"; and Bill Brown, "Science Fiction, the World's Fair, and the Prosthetics of Empire, 1910–1915."

7   I borrow the term *prosthetic territory* from Gabriel Brahm Jr. and Mark Driscoll's anthology, *Prosthetic Territories: Politics and Hypertechnologies*. I expand on the concept of the prosthetic territory later in this chapter.

8   For an elaborate statistical analysis of mortality from amputation during the nineteenth century, see Figg and Beck 458–60.

9   B. A. Watson's *A Treatise on Amputations of the Extremities and Their Complications* (1885), a 750-page compendium that proclaims itself the first "encyclopaedic monograph containing the important facts, theories, and arguments relating to amputations of the extremities and their complications" (v), includes lengthy chapters on anesthesia and antisepsis (the book is even dedicated to Lister, "the father of antiseptic surgery, whose labors mark a new era in the treatment of wounds") in addition to a survey of major surgical approaches to every conceivable type of amputation. Although Watson stresses that amputation should be used only as a last resort, he nevertheless lauds the technological advancements that enable "the modern surgeon" to perform "this operation without pain, increasing instead of diminishing the patient's chances of life and usefulness, and [shortening] the period of suffering" (99).

10   In *Death, Dissection and the Destitute*, Ruth Richardson notes the importance of bodily integrity to cultural conceptions of death and resurrection, arguing that anxieties about the spiritual effects of dismemberment fueled popular resistance to dissection throughout the nineteenth century. According to Richardson, emergent scientific imperatives violated traditional ideas about the relationship between body and soul; simply put, the concern was that the spirit could not rest in peace if the body itself was in pieces (see "The Corpse and Popular Culture" 3–29; and "The Sanctity of the Grave Asserted" 75–99). Amputees frequently buried their limbs in an effort to lay such anxieties to rest. According to American folklore, burying the limb in a straight position reduced the likelihood of a painful, or "cramped," phantom limb. For an account of Western attitudes toward limb burial since the Middle Ages, see Douglas B. Price, "Miraculous Restoration of Lost Body Parts: Relationship to the Phantom Limb Phenomenon and to Limb-Burial Superstitions and Practices."

11   Growing out of his experiences treating injured Civil War soldiers at the U.S. Army Hospital for Diseases of the Nervous System in Philadelphia, Mitchell's book gave the most complete account of nerve injuries to date—including the first extended analysis of the pathology of stumps—and became a standard text for the remainder of the century. The book represents an expansion of *Gunshot Wounds and Other Injuries of Nerves*, a detailed compilation of forty-three case studies with comparatively little theoretical apparatus that Mitchell published in 1864 with his colleagues G. Morehouse and W. W. Keen.

12   Mitchell notes that reflex actions are often accompanied by pain in the stump: "I have seen one person who has a sharp pang in the arm-stump (left) when he yawns, and others who always suffer more or less in leg-stumps (thigh) during defecation" (*Injuries* 346).

13   Victorians disagreed about where hysteria came from, alternately ascribing it to diseased reproductive organs, an imbalanced nervous system, or an ill-defined combination of the two. However, they generally agreed about what it looked like. My profile of hysteria is deliberately impressionistic, concentrating more on how stumps participated in what was by the nineteenth century a well-defined iconography than on how stumps figured into debates about hysteria's etiology. Even so, I have drawn specifically on Jean-Martin Charcot's formulation, which divides the body into "hysterogenic zones," describes stigmata in terms of sensory and motor disturbances, and coins the term *clownism* to describe the more acrobatic phases of hysterical fits. Charcot and Mitchell wrote at roughly the same time. The standard account of hysteria is Ilza Veith's *Hysteria: The History of a Disease*. See also George Frederick Drinka, *The Birth of Neurosis: Myth, Malady, and the Victorians;* Edward Shorter, *From Paralysis to Fatigue: A History of Psychosomatic Illness in the Modern Era;* and Elaine Showalter, *The Female Malady: Women, Madness, and Culture in England, 1830–1900.*

14   For a different reading of Mitchell's sexual politics, see Leslie Katz, "Flesh of His Flesh: Amputation in *Moby Dick* and S. W. Mitchell's Medical Papers." Katz argues that Mitchell distributes the problematic pathology of amputation across gendered bodies, recuperating the embattled masculinity of the dismembered man by figuring the hysterical woman as a stump.

15   Men could, of course, have hysteria. As Charcot, among others, was quick to point out, once the nervous system replaced the reproductive organs in etiological accounts of hysteria, the male body became vulnerable to the disease. Even so, hysteria was still thought of as a disease of women; to diagnose a man with hysteria was to feminize him. On male hysteria, see Shorter 117–20.

16   In this respect, Victorian medicine remained bound by binary notions of gender even as it attempted to theorize a body that was, in more ways than one, far removed from gender norms. See Thomas Laqueur's *Making Sex* for an analysis of how an ideology of sexual difference based on the notion of biological incommensurability was consolidated over the eighteenth and nineteenth centuries. Medicine's tendency to figure the pathology of amputation in terms of feminization must be seen as part of the wider movement during the second half of the nineteenth century to see "failed men"—masturbators, neurotics, and homosexuals (otherwise known as "inverts")—as perverse images of women. On the Victorian construction of sexual deviance, see Jeffrey Weeks, *Sex, Politics and Society: The Regulation of Sexuality since 1800;* and Ed Cohen, *Talk on the Wilde Side: Toward a Genealogy of a Discourse on Male Sexualities.* More recently, James Eli Adams has argued that even normative rhetorics of Victorian masculinity encoded a certain effeminacy, most characteristically in the language surrounding intellectual labor.

Adams contends that the fragility built into manliness was as productive as it was problematic. See *Dandies and Desert Saints: Styles of Victorian Manhood,* especially pp. 1–19. The amputated male body was one of many sites where Victorians generated conceptual movement—at once problematic and, as we shall see, enormously productive—by way of a strategically unstable model of gender.

17 Although Mitchell was the first to name phantom limbs as such, they were described as early as 1545 by Ambroise Paré.

18 On Lord Nelson, see Siegfried and Zimmerman 2; on Descartes, see Morris 315 n.10. Mitchell's interest in explicating the neurology of phantom limbs has lasted to this day. Books on amputation typically include a chapter on the phenomenon, and in 1981 papers presented at an international symposium on phantom and stump pain were collected into the first full-length volume on the subject. See Siegfried and Zimmerman, *Phantom and Stump Pain.*

19 Mitchell's use of spectral language to describe the neurological pathologies of stumps draws on Victorian debates about the ontological status of the spirit world. Spiritualism was immensely popular at the same time that ghosts were being debunked by the new scientific materialism, and skeptics saw mediums—usually women—as borderline hysterics at best, and patent frauds at worst. Conjuring the absent limb as a shadowy presence, Mitchell's stumps take shape as mad mediums, dangerously susceptible beings whose sensitivity to ghosts only ever proves that they have taken leave of their senses. On the medicalization of the spirit medium, see Alex Owen's chapter "Medicine, Mediumship, and Mania," in *The Darkened Room: Women, Power, and Spiritualism in Late Victorian England.*

20 Terry Castle has argued that the nineteenth-century interest in "phantasmagoria," or light shows designed to project visual images into space, functioned both to vaporize ghosts (which were exposed as the products of "spectral technologies") and to relocate them in the mind, where, Castle notes, they continue to haunt us in the form of dreams and thoughts. Phantom limbs sat neatly at the nexus of these debates about ghosts: like all good spectral technologies, they seemed real but were actually all in the amputee's head (or his stump). See "Phantasmagoria: Spectral Technology and the Metaphorics of Modern Reverie."

21 Reamputation does actually have therapeutic value. Phantom limb pain originates in irritated or traumatized nerve endings; it can sometimes be corrected by surgically resectioning the nerves or, more seriously, by reconstructing the stump itself. Even so, the use of amputation to treat phantom limbs resonates with the way it was sometimes used to treat inexplicable symptoms in the otherwise healthy limbs of women. Benjamin Brodie solved the problem of one woman's hysterical paralysis by simply cutting off the offending leg. See Shorter 126–27.

22 Similarly, James Paget argued that the body's ability to repair itself depended on injured parts being able to recapitulate a healthy organization. While a discussion of how amputation mobilized anxieties about atavistic regression (recall Dedlow's horror at being reduced to a "larval" state) is beyond the scope of this chapter, it is interesting to note that Paget saw the body's capacity for repair as inversely

proportional to its position on the evolutionary scale: only the lowest animals are capable of regenerating whole organs and limbs; more complex species can mend only local injuries. In Paget's logic, the regenerative impulse of phantom limb pain would be a sign of incipient degeneration. See *Lectures on Surgical Pathology* 119–88.

23   Mitchell's model of the phantom as a fragmented entity is curiously anticipated by Charles Dickens's *A Christmas Carol* (1843), where the Ghost of Christmas Past appears to Scrooge as a shifting vision of disparate parts: "the figure itself fluctuated in its distinctness: being now a thing with one arm, now with one leg, now with twenty legs, now a pair of legs without a head, now a head without a body: of which dissolving parts no outline would be visible in the dense gloom wherein they melted away" (43). Dickens's image of a phantom with phantom limbs—or rather of the phantom *as* phantom limbs—points to the peculiar entanglement of neurological and narrative forms in Victorian thinking about the somatic basis of selfhood.

24   Mitchell's parody of spiritualist explanations of phantom limbs takes place in the context of a more general insistence on the part of nineteenth-century medicine that so-called paranormal phenomena could always be explained away by science. Spiritualists countered efforts to discredit them by arguing that paranormal phenomena were in fact authenticated by scientific principles. See Janet Oppenheim, *The Other World: Spiritualism and Psychical Research in England, 1850–1914*. More broadly, the story draws on a set of generic conventions that had been associated with accounts of limb loss since the Middle Ages. The phantasmatic restoration of lost limbs was the subject of saints' legends and miraculous stories throughout the medieval and early modern periods. These tales, which typically feature the regeneration of a lost member with some or all of the properties of the original limb were the subject of religious and medical fascination through the mid-eighteenth century. See Douglas B. Price and Neil J. Twombly, *The Phantom Limb Phenomenon: A Medical, Folkloric, and Historical Study*.

25   Sometimes the recombination of phantom and prosthesis failed to occur, although that was very rare. James describes one case in which the phantom failed to fuse with the artificial limb: "He felt as if he had three legs in all, getting sometimes confused, in coming down stairs, between the artificial leg which he put forwards, and the imaginary one which he felt bent backwards and in danger of scraping its toes upon the steps just left behind" (3).

26   In a similar vein, Mitchell argues that prosthetics act as a visual corrective for the individual amputee, who recovers a balanced perspective by learning to look at himself differently: "When we replace the lost leg by an artificial member—which for purposes of locomotion competently supplies the place of the missing limb—such feelings as result in the notion of shortening are continually antagonized by the seeing of the foot in its position and by its fulfillment of function, while this is aided by the impressions which come to the brain from such of the remaining upper muscles as move in the act of walking, and which equally act in locomotion with the

acquired member. It is then found that by degrees the leg seems to lengthen again, until once more the foot assumes its proper place" ("Phantom Limbs" 567).

27   The optimism articulated here by James and Mitchell is at once historically specific and typical of Western writing about artificial limbs from the fifteenth century on. The fantasy of a mechanically perfect substitute for lost limbs had animated Swiss, French, and German inventors for centuries by the time nineteenth-century advances in surgery and prosthetic technology made the dream realizable. More particularly, late-eighteenth- and early-nineteenth-century advances in German surgery, especially in the related arts of amputation and facial reconstruction, laid the groundwork for the idea that an amputee could be remade. Carl Ferdinand von Graefe (1787–1840) was the single most important figure in forging this symbolic and technical synthesis. Not only was he the father of plastic surgery (he even coined the term *rhinoplasty*) and a fantastically successful amputator of limbs (in the era before antisepsis and anesthesia, his patients had a phenomenally low rate of infection and high rate of survival), he was also a vocal proponent of the idea that surgery must do its utmost to reconstruct lost body parts—whether by crafting new noses from remaining flesh or shaping healthy, weight-bearing stumps capable of wearing artificial limbs. The extent to which British and especially American-made limbs articulated an ideal of reconstruction during the latter half of the century is the extent to which surgeons and limb makers assimilated the vision von Graefe articulated so forcefully nearly half a century before. On von Graefe, see Blair O. Rogers, "Carl Ferdinand von Graefe." On early limbs, see Reed Benhamou, "The Artificial Limb in Preindustrial France."

28   The laborious turn of prosthetic language reflects the fact that it was addressed specifically to working-class amputees. Although soldiers were the principal subjects of Victorian medical writing about amputation, the discourse of prosthesis—which was developed most fully by those who were making and selling limbs—was oriented almost entirely around the advantages that artificial limbs offer the manual laborer. The reasons for this are several: although soldiers were certainly the most visible and sympathetic images of dismemberment during the nineteenth century, there was a large and ever-expanding population of mutilated working men. More to the point: veterans had their limbs subsidized by the state in both Britain and America, while workingmen typically had to purchase, maintain, and replace their own. As a consequence, limb makers in both countries targeted the private citizen, competing for control of this new market by appealing to the physical needs of men whose livelihood depended on returning to work. Women are almost wholly absent from the literature of prosthesis (an exception is A. A. Marks, who included a few testimonials from housewives in his mail-order catalog and marketed women's limbs). Professional men are simply represented in terms that echo those more energetically applied to working-class men.

29   For an analysis of the prosthetic logic of Victorian thinking about manufacture, see Tamara Ketabgian, "The Human Prosthesis: Workers and Machines in the Victorian Industrial Scene."

30   Manufacturers of artificial limbs relied heavily on personal testimonials to endorse their products. Their catalogs reprinted letters from customers detailing all the things their limbs enabled them to do, and even reproduced photos of wearers at work and at play. The bulk of the testimonials quoted here are drawn from the mail-order catalogs of A. A. Marks, one of the most prominent limb makers in the world during the latter half of the nineteenth century. Marks had a global reputation, and his ever-thickening catalogs contained hundreds of testimonials from satisfied customers all over the world. Other makers—Palmer, Ferris, Kimball, and Rowley, to name a few—printed short pamphlets and booklets that replicated Marks's marketing strategy on a much smaller scale. Weir Mitchell preferred Kimball limbs.

31   Poe wrote this story well before the major advances in nineteenth-century prosthetics, and his concern about mechanization is understandable given the state of artificial limb technology when he was writing. What is perhaps most interesting about Poe's story, however, is how it anticipates the kinds of complications really well-made limbs would cause for conceptions of personhood. The story basically projects the logic of prosthesis past its own technological moment; it is in many ways about a half century ahead of itself.

32   The word *counterfeit* is used repeatedly to describe an effective imitation of actual limbs; advertisers, doctors, and wearers all joined in coining the term.

33   Manufacturers argued that the extra cost would eventually save the amputee a great deal of money and embarrassment. In addition to concealing the fact of the amputee's loss, so that he no longer had to appear before the public with clattering and inefficient limbs, state-of-the-art legs cost almost nothing to maintain. In America at the turn of the century, wearers reported spending anywhere from five to twenty-five dollars annually to repair the fragile ankle joints in wooden legs, an expense that was eradicated by limbs that substituted a flexible rubber foot for an elaborately mechanized joint. Although both Marks and Rowley required a substantial down payment, both made it possible for limbs to be bought by installments.

34   The rubber foot was invented by A. A. Marks in 1861 and patented in 1863. He continued to improve on the basic model throughout the rest of the century, patenting a foot with laminated toes in 1880, and adding a spring mattress for additional resiliency in 1895. As of 1888, more than eight thousand rubber feet were being worn worldwide, and as of 1903, sixteen thousand were in use, a fact Marks pointed to as evidence of their superiority to other makes. By the end of the century other manufacturers were marketing variations on the basic theme; in 1886, J. F. Rowley, who invented the custom-molded wax socket and also patented special ball-bearing knee joints, patented a rubber foot with an internal hinge connecting it to the core of the artificial leg.

35   Like the term *counterfeit*, the word *substitute* was a synonym for prosthesis at all levels of the discourse. *Appleton's Journal* simply spells out the association that is everywhere else assumed—that what is being substituted is nature itself.

36   A. A. Marks reprinted the song of the cork leg in the first and second editions of his pamphlet on artificial limbs, noting that to the best of his knowledge, cork legs were purely mythical creations.

37   Rowley's chapter on the "Man Re-built" includes photos of "legless athletes." Reprinting a list of the records set by wearers of his legs, Rowley recounted the process by which wearer and manufacturer both cashed in on the rebuilt body. Rowley "persistently advertised legless athletes as evidence of the superiority of our artificial leg," and these athletes in turn sold themselves to the highest bidder: "The numerous individuals whom we have advertised, have endeavored to realize on our advertising, by embarking in the business themselves or entering the employ of some firm which makes slip-socket and ankle jointed legs, until more than one-half of the leg salesmen and almost the entire crop of amateur leg makers of the middle west have been either advertised by or [have] worked for J. F. Rowley" (112).

38   In reading Baum's story as a twentieth-century extension of Victorian logics of prosthesis, I do not mean to discount the tremendous impact of World War I on ideas about dismemberment. By producing unprecedented numbers of amputees, the Great War made mutilation more visible than it had ever been before. As such, it not only heightened political and social sensitivity to disability in general, but also placed a great deal of pressure on models of manliness and national identity as more and more soldiers came home safe but not sound. Histories of mutilation and orthopedics tend to locate World War I as the moment when dismemberment entered technological and conceptual modernity, arguing that the war forced orthopedics to come into its own by generating a widespread need for durable, lightweight limbs that were both functional and aesthetic. This chapter complicates that claim: as we have seen, the pressure to develop functional, practically invisible limbs and the pressure to conceptualize a masculinity that could accommodate dismemberment and prosthesis originated during the nineteenth century, and both were associated with distinctly Victorian anxieties about the impact of medical, military, and industrial modernity on men's gender identity. On the place of orthopedics in modern medicine, see Roger Cooter, *Surgery and Society in Peace and War: Orthopaedics and the Organization of Modern Medicine, 1880–1948.*

39   For an analysis of the gender politics of the "Ozian" fantasy of a detachable, indestructible identity, see Stuart Culver's "Growing Up in Oz."

40   Freud himself was much troubled by his own prosthesis, a rubber jaw installed in 1923 to replace the one he lost to cancer. Describing himself as waging a "small-scale war . . . with a refractory piece of equipment," he understood prosthetics as the sign of a necessary, but always problematic, series of tensions between fallible bodies and the innumerable gadgets devised to enhance and perfect them. The "substitute . . . which tries to be and yet cannot be the self . . . is a problem which arises even in the case of spectacles, false teeth and wigs, but not so insistently as in the case of a prosthesis" (Freud, *Letters* 137).

41   The anthology develops the term *prosthetic territory* from Mark Wigley's essay "Prosthetic Theory: The Disciplining of Architecture." The author cites Wigley's

definition of prosthesis and adapts it thus: "A 'prosthesis' can be defined as a 'foreign element that reconstructs that which cannot stand up on its own, at once propping up and extending its host. The prosthesis is always structural, establishing the place it appears to add to.' When the border between the 'foreign' and the 'native'—the cultural and the natural, the political and the cultural, the social and the political—can no longer readily be justified or perhaps even maintained, we have entered 'prosthetic territory'" (Brahm and Driscoll 1–2).

42   A notable exception is David Wills's elegant *Prosthesis,* which puts the concept through a range of intricate philosophical, historical, and etymological paces without ever losing sight of its material dimensions: the book is framed in large part as an effort to come to grips with the emotional and ontological complexities of his own father's wooden leg.

4. MONSTERS, MATERIALS, METHODS

1   Many of these can still be seen. The Royal College of Surgeons at Lincoln's Inn Fields, London, houses the Hunterian collection, which contains, among other anomalies, the tallest articulated skeleton on record, that of Charles Byrne, the eight-foot-four-inch-tall "Irish Giant." Byrne's bones, acquired illegally by Hunter in 1783, stand next to those of Caroline Crachami, the twenty-inch-tall "Sicilian Fairy," who died during a show tour in 1824. The Mutter Museum at the Philadelphia College of Physicians houses the second-tallest articulated skeleton in the world along with the conjoined liver of Chang and Eng.

2   My argument here is indebted to Catherine Gallagher's observation that when it comes to Victorian patterns of meaning making, the socially marginal is often symbolically central. See "The Body versus the Social Body in the Works of Thomas Malthus and Henry Mayhew." Most work on the history of monstrosity associates it with issues of identity. Classics such as Leslie Fiedler's *Freaks: Myths and Images of the Secret Self* read the monster as a virtually timeless challenge to the concept of personhood, while more recent studies such as Robert Bogdan's *Freak Show: Presenting Human Oddities for Amusement and Profit* and Rosemarie Garland Thomson's anthology *Freakery: Cultural Spectacles of the Extraordinary Body* draw more precise connections between the monsters of the nineteenth and twentieth centuries and modern ideological patterns.

3   *Monster* comes from the Latin *monstrare,* which means "to warn, show, or sign." *Monstrare* is the root of the verb *demonstrate.*

4   In contrast with the previous chapters, this chapter concentrates less on medical treatments of deformity than on popular attitudes toward and representations of disfigurement. Although medicine was interested in the monster, as evidenced by the flowering of teratology and embryology during this period, the monster was thoroughly medicalized only at the end of the century, when endocrinology and the revival of Mendelian genetics made it possible to comprehend physical anom-

aly in chemical terms. Up to that point, medical writing about monstrosity was largely descriptive, emphasizing classification over intervention, observation over cure. Teratology, or the science of monsters, was formalized in 1832 by Geoffroy Saint-Hilaire's *Histoire générale et particulière des anomalies de l'organisation chez l'homme et les animaux*. As a science, it was far more concerned with taxonomy and theory than with experimentation; in practice, doctors were basically helpless before the spectacle of human defect, incapable of arresting its progress or easing its pains. The freak show was where Victorians thought the monster most inventively; the outrageous logics generated there tended to absorb more sober, scientific formulations. Indeed, in many ways Victorian medicine functioned as an adjunct to the freak show—sideshow circulars frequently used excerpts from medical reports on specific monsters to bolster their claims to veracity. On nineteenth-century exhibitionary culture, see Richard Altick, *The Shows of London;* Thomas Richards, *The Commodity Culture of Victorian England;* and Tony Bennett, "The Exhibitionary Complex," in *The Birth of the Museum: History, Theory, Politics.*

5 For a thorough account of Tom Thumb's trips to London, see Fitzsimons, *Barnum in London.* The English reception of Barnum's freaks was profoundly different from the American one. As Neil Harris shows in *Humbug: The Art of P. T. Barnum,* the American people saw the freak show as a chance to constitute itself as a sophisticated audience that was capable of differentiating between authentic shows and the humbuggery that was so central to Barnumesque display. British hostility toward Barnum's antics reached its peak when Barnum published his autobiography in 1855. Barnum's *Life* contains a long chapter on how he hoodwinked the English public into paying millions to admire a dwarf who was no more unusual, at least physically, than England's own little people. For British reactions to the *Life,* see "Barnum"; "The Great American Humbug"; and "Revelations of a Showman," reviews printed by *Fraser's, Tait's,* and *Blackwood's,* respectively.

6 In this respect, monsters were part of a much larger project of cultural re-visioning. According to Jonathan Crary, the nineteenth century saw a revolution in visual technology that reconstituted vision itself. I read the monster as one of the long series of optical instruments (cameras, kaleidoscopes, stereoscopes, magic lanterns, etc.) that Crary argues produced a new kind of observer, an individual whose perceptions are uniquely suited to "a constellation of new events, forces and institutions that together are loosely and perhaps tautologically definable as 'modernity'" (9). See *Techniques of the Observer: On Vision and Modernity in the Nineteenth Century.* See also Carol T. Christ and John O. Jordan's anthology, *Victorian Literature and the Victorian Visual Imagination.*

7 On Chang and Eng, see Fiedler 204–5, 213–18.

8 See Stallybrass and White 119–20 on Wordsworth. Bennett's discussion of Wordsworth explicitly builds on Stallybrass and White's (86). The lines on Bartholomew Fair have also made their way into Richard Altick's *Shows of London* (36) and James Twitchell's *Carnival Culture: The Trashing of Taste in America.*

9   I should note here that Wordsworth's lines establish an analogy between monsters and nonwhite people that has historically been characteristic of logics of deformity. I return to the issue of race later in this chapter.

10   Mark Seltzer develops the concept of miscegenation in *Bodies and Machines,* using it as a metaphor for the unsightly results of breeding disparate cultural forms: miscegenation is a standard gesture of machine culture, describing "the erosion of the boundaries that divide persons and things, labor and nature, what counts as an agent and what doesn't. . . . [S]uch an erosion of boundaries immediately evokes the melodramas of uncertain agency everywhere rehearsed in the work of dividing 'nature' from 'culture'" (21). This notion takes on a strikingly literal feel when human reproduction is the scene of categorical transgression, and when an unassimilable monster is the result.

11   Neil Harris's *Humbug* and A. H. Saxon's *P. T. Barnum* provide excellent accounts of Barnum's career. Kunhardt's *P. T. Barnum* supplies a fascinating pictorial history of the American Museum and the living curiosities that resided there.

12   Dickens was publishing *The Old Curiosity Shop* (1840–41) as Barnum was assembling his. Like Barnum, Dickens was more invested in his living curiosities than in his inanimate ones, stocking the story with two tiny heroines (Nell and the Marchioness), an evil dwarf (Quilp), and a bizarre cast of minor characters, including a lady with no arms or legs and a weak-kneed giant. Dickens was fascinated by freaks; he even made a special visit to Barnum's museum during his American tour.

13   Barnum was instrumental in popularizing natural history, making specimens from around the world available to the public. See John Rickards Betts, "P. T. Barnum and the Popularization of Natural History."

14   Seltzer develops the idea of "drawing into relation" throughout *Bodies and Machines.* See Miller's essay "The Late Jane Austen" for "conceptual crossovers," and Grossberg's *We Gotta Get out of This Place* for an elaborate defense of this model of interdisciplinary thought.

15   I refer here to the semiotics of spectacle that critics such as Jean Baudrillard and Guy Debord see as central to consumer culture. In *The Commodity Culture of Victorian England,* Thomas Richards locates the originary moment of spectacle in the Great Exhibition of 1851. This chapter builds on Richards's argument, treating the freak show as part of that moment of spectacular genesis.

16   Even teratology, the new science of monsters, could not explain them. Unable to develop a satisfying theory for the causes of birth defects, let alone a cure, medicine concentrated on classification and description. As the teratologist Geoffroy Saint-Hilaire wrote, "Monsters are not sports of nature; their organization is subject to rules, to rigorously defined laws, and these rules, these laws, are identical with those that regulate the animal series; in a word, monsters are also normal beings; or rather, there are no monsters, and nature is one whole" (quoted in Oppenheimer 147). As if to say that conceptual control could effect cure, science fantasized about managing monstrosity by defining it away. On nineteenth-century efforts to dis-

cover a physiological basis for birth defects, see Jane Oppenheimer, "Some Historical Relationships between Teratology and Experimental Embryology."

17 B. A. Morel offered the first fully formulated theory of degeneration in his 1857 *Traité des Dégénérescences*, which crystallized a concept that would obsess British, American, and Continental thinking well into the twentieth century. For a cultural history of degeneration, see Daniel Pick, *Faces of Degeneration: A European Disorder, c. 1848–1918*.

18 Freak shows frequently capitalized on Darwinian ideas and a growing popular awareness of foreign cultures by presenting exotic people as freaks, and by showing nonwhites as missing links, displaced signs of more primitive evolutionary times. Most commonly, missing links were retarded dwarves—after William Henry Johnson (Zip), the most celebrated of these anachronistic figures were Maximo and Bartola, microcephalic Salvadoran dwarves who were billed as "The Last of the Ancient Aztecs" (on the Aztec children, see Bogdan 127–34; on Zip, see Bogdan 134–42). Much of the work on the Victorian freak show has centered on these figures, using them to historicize the timeless logic of objectification embodied in the freak show. As the story goes, the freak show has always been a scene of othering, a mechanism for consolidating the spectator's sense of herself as "normal" by staging an undeniable contrast between the misshapen body on display and the viewer's own relatively unremarkable one (Bogdan, Grosz, Fiedler). During the nineteenth century, critics have argued, freak shows took on just the sort of historically specific contours one might expect—in an age of exploration, expansion, and increasing curiosity about "savage" people, for example, the freak show became a distinctly imperial carnival, a fabulous showcase for the freakishness of race itself. This spectacular racism was but one dimension of the freak show, however. This chapter concentrates on moments when monsters figured less as exotic others than as models of a new, improved self.

19 On the place of monstrosity in nineteenth-century theories of evolution, see Evelleen Richards, "A Political Anatomy of Monsters, Hopeful and Otherwise: Teratogeny, Transcendentalism, and Evolutionary Theorizing."

20 Unlike artificial legs, prosthetic hands were notoriously inferior to the parts they replaced. Prosthetic technology could imitate gross motor movements of the lower extremities, but not the fine coordinations of the upper body.

21 On carnival as the scene of rampant symbolic inversion, see Mikhail Bakhtin, *Rabelais and His World*. On the centrality of carnivalesque inversion to nineteenth-century structures of imagining, see Stallybrass and White, *The Politics and Poetics of Transgression*, especially the chapters on the city, the family, and the hysteric.

AFTERWORD

1 For a sampling of literary, historical, and theoretical work on the subject, see Richard Altick, *The Shows of London;* Robert Bogdan, *Freak Show: Presenting Human Oddities for Amusement and Profit;* Jeffrey Jerome Cohen's anthology, *Mon-*

ster Theory: Reading Culture; Marie-Hélène Huet, *Monstrous Imagination;* Rosemarie Garland Thomson's collection, *Freakery: Cultural Spectacles of the Extraordinary Body;* and Dennis Todd, *Imagining Monsters: Miscreations of the Self in Eighteenth-Century England.*

2 For psychoanalytic accounts of monstrosity, see Elisabeth Grosz, "Intolerable Ambiguity: Freaks as/at the Limit"; and Leslie Fiedler, *Freaks: Myths and Images of the Secret Self.*

3 For postcolonial work, see Sander Gilman, "Black Bodies, White Bodies"; and Bernth Lindfors, "Ethnological Show Business: Footlighting the Dark Continent."

4 In the late 1970s and early 1980s, feminist criticism embraced the monster as the symbol of corrupt social forms and feminist resistance to these forms. Where Dorothy Dinnerstein discussed the monstrousness of gender relations under patriarchy in *The Mermaid and the Minotaur: Sexual Arrangements and Human Malaise,* and Barbara Johnson drew on Dinnerstein and *Frankenstein* to describe the "monstrousness" of parenthood in "My Monster, My Self," Nina Auerbach's *Woman and the Demon: The Life of a Victorian Myth* and Sandra Gilbert and Susan Gubar's *The Madwoman in the Attic: The Woman Writer and the Nineteenth-Century Literary Imagination* showed how the historic demonization of women both diminishes them and provides the source of a special female power. Mary Russo's *Female Grotesque: Risk, Excess, and Modernity* is the most recent addition to this genre.

5 Rosemarie Garland Thomson's *Extraordinary Bodies: Figuring Physical Disability in American Culture and Literature* is a major study in this new field.

6 Bakhtin's concept of carnival has been central to cultural theory since Peter Stallybrass and Allon White invoked it in their pathbreaking work *The Politics and Poetics of Transgression.* Since then, a wide range of work has explored the so-called carnivalesque dimensions of modern culture. For a sampling, see Michael André Bernstein, *Bitter Carnival: Ressentiment and the Abject Hero;* Mary Russo, *The Female Grotesque;* and James Twitchell, *Carnival Culture.*

7 Michael Bérubé, Stanley Fish, John Guillory, Lawrence Grossberg, Cary Nelson, Bruce Robbins, Andrew Ross, and David Simpson are some of the best-known contributors to this discussion.

8 For representative articulations of cultural studies's mission and its related reluctance to define itself, see Richard Johnson, "What Is Cultural Studies Anyway?" and the introduction to *Cultural Studies,* edited by Grossberg, Nelson, and Treichler.

9 For arguments on either side of this question, see Michael Bérubé, *Public Access: Literary Theory and American Cultural Politics;* and Stanley Fish, *Professional Correctness: Literary Studies and Political Change.* Bérubé's more recent *The Employment of English: Theory, Jobs, and the Future of Literary Studies* extends both his earlier arguments and his argument with Fish about the value of cultural studies.

Acton, William. *Prostitution; Considered in Its Moral, Social, and Sanitary Aspects in London and Other Large Cities and Garrison Towns with Proposals for the Control and Prevention of Its Attendant Evils.* 1857. London: Frank Cass, 1972.

Adams, James Eli. *Dandies and Desert Saints: Styles of Victorian Manhood.* Ithaca: Cornell UP, 1995.

Alcott, Louisa May. *Hospital Sketches.* 1863. Boston: Applewood, 1986.

Altick, Richard Daniel. *The Shows of London.* Cambridge: Belknap, 1978.

Anderson, Amanda. *Tainted Souls and Painted Faces: The Rhetoric of Fallenness in Victorian Culture.* Ithaca: Cornell UP, 1993.

Anderson, Benedict. *Imagined Communities: Reflections on the Origin and Spread of Nationalism.* London: Verso, 1983.

Arlidge, J. T. *The Hygiene Diseases and Mortality of Occupations.* London: Percival, 1892.

Armstrong, Nancy. *Desire and Domestic Fiction: A Political History of the Novel.* New York: Oxford UP, 1987.

Arnold, David. *Colonizing the Body: State Medicine and Disease in Nineteenth-Century India.* Berkeley: U California P, 1993.

—, ed. *Imperial Medicine and Indigenous Societies.* Manchester: Manchester UP, 1988.

Ashcroft, Bill, Gareth Griffiths, and Helen Tiffin, eds. *The Postcolonial Studies Reader.* London: Routledge, 1992.

Auerbach, Nina. *Communities of Women: An Idea in Fiction.* Cambridge: Harvard UP, 1978.

—. *Woman and the Demon: The Life of a Victorian Myth.* Cambridge: Harvard UP, 1982.

Bailin, Miriam. *The Sickroom in Victorian Fiction: The Art of Being Ill.* New York: Cambridge UP, 1994.

Bain, Alexander. *The Emotions and the Will.* London: John W. Parker, 1859.

—. *Mind and Body: The Theories of Their Relation.* London: Henry S. King, 1873.

Bakhtin, Mikhail. *Rabelais and His World.* Trans. Hélène Iswolsky. Bloomington: Indiana UP, 1984.

Banks, W. Mitchell. "On Free Removal of Mammary Cancer, with Extirpation of the Axillary Glands as a Necessary Accompaniment." *British Medical Journal* 2 (1882): 1138–41. (Reprinted in Robbins, *Silvergirl's Surgery: The Breast,* 69–71).

"Barnum." *Fraser's Magazine* 51 (February 1855): 213–23.

Barnum, P. T. *The Life of P. T. Barnum.* New York: Redfield, 1855.

Bauerlein, Mark. *Literary Criticism: An Autopsy.* Philadelphia: U Pennsylvania P, 1997.

Baum, L. Frank. *The Tin Woodman of Oz.* Chicago: Rand McNally, 1918.

Beer, Gillian. *Darwin's Plots: Evolutionary Narrative in Darwin, George Eliot, and Nineteenth-Century Fiction.* London: Routledge and Kegan Paul, 1983.

Benhamou, Reed. "The Artificial Limb in Preindustrial France." *Technology & Culture* 35 (October 1994): 835–45.

Benison, Saul. Preface to Thackrah, *The Effects of Arts, Trades, and Professions on Health and Longevity.*

Bennett, Tony. *The Birth of the Museum: History, Theory, Politics.* New York: Routledge, 1995.

Benson, John A. *Asiatic Cholera: Its Genesis, Etiological Factors, Clinical History, Pathology, and Treatment.* Chicago: J. Harrison White, 1893.

Bernstein, Michael André. *Bitter Carnival: Ressentiment and the Abject Hero.* Princeton: Princeton UP, 1992.

Bérubé, Michael. *The Employment of English: Theory, Jobs, and the Future of Literary Studies.* New York: New York UP, 1998.

—. *Public Access: Literary Theory and American Cultural Politics.* London: Verso, 1994.

Betts, John Rickards. "P. T. Barnum and the Popularization of Natural History." *Journal of the History of Ideas* 20 (1959): 353–68.

Birkett, John. *The Diseases of the Breast, and Their Treatment.* London: Longman, Brown, Green, and Longmans, 1850.

Bogdan, Robert. *Freak Show: Presenting Human Oddities for Amusement and Profit.* Chicago: U Chicago P, 1988.

Bolt, Christine. *Victorian Attitudes to Race.* London: Routledge and Kegan Paul, 1971.

Booth, Charles. *Labour and Life of the People in London.* London: Macmillan, 1902–4.

Bordo, Susan. *Unbearable Weight: Feminism, Western Culture, and the Body.* Berkeley: U California P, 1993.

Bourdelais, Patrice, and André Dodin. *Visages du Cholera.* Paris: Belin, 1987.

Bourdieu, Pierre. *Distinction: A Social Critique of the Judgement of Taste.* Trans. Richard Nice. Cambridge: Harvard UP, 1984.

Bourke, Joanna. *Dismembering the Male: Men's Bodies, Britain and the Great War.* Chicago: U Chicago P, 1996.

Bowlby, Rachel. *Just Looking: Consumer Culture in Dreiser, Gissing, and Zola.* New York: Methuen, 1985.

Brahm, Gabriel Jr., and Mark Driscoll, eds. *Prosthetic Territories: Politics and Hypertechnologies.* Boulder: Westview, 1995.

Brantlinger, Patrick. *Crusoe's Footprints: Cultural Studies in Britain and America.* New York: Routledge, 1990.

Brodie, Benjamin. *Mind and Matter; or, Physiological Inquiries.* New York: G. P. Putnam, 1857.

Brown, Bill. "Science Fiction, the World's Fair, and the Prosthetics of Empire, 1910–1915." In *Cultures of United States Imperialism,* ed. Amy Kaplan and Donald E. Pease, 129–63. Durham: Duke UP, 1993.

Brown, Gillian. "Anorexia, Humanism, and Feminism." *Yale Journal of Criticism* 5 (Fall 1991): 189–215.

Brown, John. *Rab and His Friends.* Boston: Ticknor and Fields, 1859.

Browne, Matthew. "The Deformed and the Stricken." *Good Words* 7 (1866): 737–40.

Bryant, Thomas. *The Diseases of the Breast.* London: Cassell, 1887.

Brydon, Diana. "The White Inuit Speaks: Contamination as Literary Strategy." In *Past the Last Post: Theorizing Postcolonialism and Post-modernism,* ed. Ian Adam and Helen Tiffin, 191–203. Calgary: U Calgary P, 1990.

Burnett, James Compton. *Tumours of the Breast, and Their Treatment and Cure by Medicines.* London: Epps, 1888.

Burney, Fanny. "A Mastectomy." In *Selected Letters and Journals*. Ed. Joyce Hemlow. New York: Oxford UP, 1986.

Butter, J. "Practical Observations on the Compression of Cancerous Breasts." *Edinburgh Medical and Surgical Journal* 14 (1818): 498–507. (Reprinted in Robbins, *Silvergirl's Surgery: The Breast*, 29–31.)

Bynum, W. F. *Science and the Practice of Medicine in the Nineteenth Century*. Cambridge: Cambridge UP, 1994.

Carlyle, Thomas. *Past and Present*. 1843. Boston: Houghton Mifflin, 1965.

—. *Sartor Resartus*. 1831. London: Dent, 1973.

Carroll, Lewis. *Through the Looking-Glass and What Alice Found There*. 1872. New York: Morrow, 1993.

Castle, Terry. "Phantasmagoria: Spectral Technology and the Metaphorics of Modern Reverie." *Critical Inquiry* 15, no. 1 (autumn 1988): 26–61.

Chadwick, Edwin. *Report on the Sanitary Condition of the Labouring Population of Great Britain*. 1842. Edinburgh: Edinburgh UP, 1965.

"Cholera Gossip." *Fraser's Magazine* 40 (1849): 702–11.

Christ, Carol T., and John O. Jordan, eds. *Victorian Literature and the Victorian Visual Imagination*. Berkeley: U California P, 1995.

Cixous, Hélène, and Catherine Clément. *The Newly Born Woman*. Trans. Betsy Wing. Minneapolis: U Minnesota P, 1986.

Cobbe, Francis Power. "Criminals, Idiots, Women, and Minors" (1868). In *"Criminals, Idiots, Women, and Minors": Nineteenth-Century Writing by Women on Women*, ed. Susan Hamilton, 108–31.

Peterborough, Ontario: Broadview, 1995.

Cohen, Ed. *Talk on the Wilde Side: Toward a Genealogy of a Discourse on Male Sexualities*. New York: Routledge, 1993.

Cohen, Jeffrey Jerome, ed. *Monster Theory: Reading Culture*. Minneapolis: U Minnesota P, 1996.

Collins, Wilkie. *Poor Miss Finch*. 1872. New York: Collier, 1876.

"The Contagious Character of Cholera." *Fraser's Magazine* 6 (1832): 119–23.

Cooper, William A. "The History of the Radical Mastectomy." *Annals of Medical History* 3 (1941): 36–54.

Cooter, Roger. *Surgery and Society in Peace and War: Orthopaedics and the Organization of Modern Medicine, 1880–1948*. Houndmills, Basingstoke, Hampshire, and London: Macmillan, 1993.

Costello, Dudley. "Monsters." *Household Words* 14 (1856): 498–504.

Cotton, Richard Payne. *The Nature, Symptoms and Treatment of Consumption*. London: John Churchill, 1852.

Coventry, C. B. *Epidemic Cholera: Its History, Causes, Pathology, and Treatment*. Buffalo: Geo. H. Derby, 1849.

Crary, Jonathan. *Techniques of the Observer: On Vision and Modernity in the Nineteenth Century*. Cambridge: MIT P, 1990.

Crawford, T. S. *A History of the Umbrella*. New York: Taplinger, 1970.

Creighton, Charles. *Contributions to the Physiology and Pathology of the Breast and Its Lymphatic Glands*. London: Macmillan, 1878.

—. *A History of Epidemics in Britain*. 2 vols. 1891. London: Frank Cass, 1965.

Crosby, Christina. "Reading the Victorians." *Victorian Studies* 36 (fall 1992): 63–74.

Cruikshank, George. "Born a Genius and Born a Dwarf" (1847). In *Comick Almanack*, Thackeray, Albert Smith, Gilbert A. Beckett, The Brothers Mayhew, 162. London: Hotten, 1853.

—. "John Bull Among the Lilliputians" (1847). In Thackeray, Smith, Beckett, and Mayhew, *Comick Almanack*, 155.

Culver, Stuart. "Growing Up in Oz." *American Literary History* 4, no. 4 (winter 1992): 607–28.

Darwin, Charles. *The Origin of Species.* 1859. Harmondsworth: Penguin, 1985.

Deaver, John B., and Joseph McFarland. *The Breast: Its Anomalies, Its Diseases, and Their Treatment.* Philadelphia: Blakiston's Son, 1917.

"The Deformed and Their Mental Characteristics." *Living Age* 72 (1862): 393–96.

"The Deformito-mania." *Punch* 3 (1848): 90.

Delaporte, François. *Disease and Civilization: The Cholera in Paris, 1832.* Cambridge, MIT P, 1986.

Dickens, Charles. *A Christmas Carol.* 1843. Harmondsworth: Penguin, 1984.

—. *David Copperfield.* 1849–50. Harmondsworth: Penguin, 1985.

—. *Dombey and Son.* 1844–46. Harmondsworth: Penguin, 1985.

—. *Hard Times.* 1854. New York: Methuen, 1961.

—. *Little Dorrit.* 1855–57. Harmondsworth: Penguin, 1985.

—. *Our Mutual Friend.* 1864–65. Oxford: Oxford UP, 1989.

—. *Pickwick Papers.* 1836–37. New York: New American Library, 1964.

—. "Please to Leave Your Umbrella." *Household Words* 17 (1858): 457–59.

Dickens, Charles, and Mark Lemon. "A Paper-Mill." *Household Words* 1 (1850): 529–31.

Dinnerstein, Dorothy. *The Mermaid and the Minotaur: Sexual Arrangements and Human Malaise.* New York: Harper and Row, 1976.

Drinka, George Frederick. *The Birth of Neurosis: Myth, Malady, and the Victorians.* New York: Simon and Schuster, 1984.

"A Drop of London Water." *Punch* 18 (1850): 188.

Dubos, René, and Jean Dubos. *The White Plague: Tuberculosis, Man and Society.* Boston: Little, Brown, 1952.

Durey, Michael. *The Return of the Plague: British Society and the Cholera 1831–32.* Dublin: Gill and Macmillan Humanities P, 1979.

During, Simon. "Postmodernism or Postcolonialism Today." *Textual Practice* 1, no. 1 (spring 1987): 32–47.

Ehrenreich, Barbara, and Deirdre English. *Complaints and Disorders: The Sexual Politics of Sickness.* New York: Feminist P, 1973.

Eliot, George. *Adam Bede.* 1859. New York: New American Library, 1981.

—. *Middlemarch.* 1871–72. New York: Norton, 1977.

Engels, Friedrich. *The Condition of the Working Class in England.* 1845. New York: Oxford UP, 1993.

Epstein, Julia. *The Iron Pen: Frances Burney and the Politics of Women's Writing.* Madison: U Wisconsin P, 1989.

Erichsen, John. *The Science and Art of Surgery: A Treatise on Surgical Injuries, Diseases, and Operations.* Philadelphia: Blanchard and Lea, 1854.

Evans, Richard J. *Death in Hamburg: Society and Politics in the Cholera Years, 1830–1910.* Oxford: Clarendon, 1987.

Fiedler, Leslie A. *Freaks: Myths and Images*

of the Secret Self. New York: Simon and Schuster, 1978.

Figg, Laurann, and Jane Farrell Beck. "Amputation in the Civil War: Physical and Social Dimensions." *Journal of the History of Medicine and Allied Sciences* 48 (1993): 454–75.

Fish, Stanley. *Professional Correctness: Literary Studies and Political Change.* New York: Clarendon, 1995.

Fitzsimons, Raymund. *Barnum in London.* New York: St. Martin's, 1970.

Ford, Henry. *My Life and Work.* New York: Doubleday, 1922.

Foucault, Michel. *Discipline and Punish: The Birth of the Prison.* Trans. Alan Sheridan. New York: Pantheon, 1977.

—. *The History of Sexuality.* Vol. 1. Trans. Robert Hurley. New York: Vintage, 1980.

Fraser, W. Hamish. *The Coming of the Mass Market, 1850–1914.* Hamden, Conn.: Archon, 1981.

Freud, Sigmund. *Civilization and Its Discontents.* 1930. Trans. James Strachey. New York: Norton, 1961.

—. *Sigmund Freud and Lou Andreas-Salomé: Letters.* Ed. Ernst Pfeiffer. Trans. William and Elaine Robson Scott. New York: Harcourt, Brace, Jovanovich, 1972.

Fryer, Judith. "'The Body in Pain' in Thomas Eakins' *Agnew Clinic.*" *Michigan Quarterly Review* 30, no. 1 (winter 1991): 191–209.

Fuss, Diana. *Essentially Speaking: Feminism, Nature and Difference.* New York: Routledge, 1989.

Gagnier, Regina. *Subjectivities: A History of Self-Representation in Britain, 1832–1920.* New York: Oxford UP, 1991.

Gallagher, Catherine. "The Bio-Economics of *Our Mutual Friend.*" In

Fragments for a History of the Human Body, ed. Michel Feher, Ramona Naddaff, and Nadia Tazi, 345–65. Cambridge: MIT P, 1989.

—. "The Body versus the Social Body in the Works of Thomas Malthus and Henry Mayhew." *Representations* 14 (spring 1986): 83–106.

Gardner, Brian. *The East India Company: A History.* New York: McCall, 1971.

Gaskell, Elizabeth. *North and South.* 1855. Harmondsworth: Penguin, 1986.

Gaskell, Peter. *Artisans and Machinery: The Moral and Physical Condition of the Manufacturing Population Considered with Reference to Mechanical Substitutes for Human Labor.* 1836. London: Frank Cass, 1968.

Gavin, Hector. *Sanitary Ramblings: Being Sketches and Illustrations, of Bethnal Green.* 1848. London: Frank Cass, 1971.

Gibbs-Smith, C. H. *The Great Exhibition of 1851: A Commemorative Album.* London: Her Majesty's Stationery Office, 1950.

Gilbert, Sandra M., and Susan Gubar. *The Madwoman in the Attic: The Woman Writer and the Nineteenth-Century Literary Imagination.* New Haven: Yale UP, 1979.

Gilman, Sander L. "Black Bodies, White Bodies: Toward an Iconography of Female Sexuality in Late Nineteenth-Century Art, Medicine, and Literature." *Critical Inquiry* 12 (autumn 1985): 204–42.

—. *Difference and Pathology: Stereotypes of Sexuality, Race, and Madness.* Ithaca: Cornell UP, 1985.

—. *Disease and Representation: Images of Illness from Madness to AIDS.* Ithaca: Cornell UP, 1988.

—. "On the Nexus of Blackness and Madness." In Gilman, *Difference and Pathology*, 131–49.

—. *Seeing the Insane.* New York: J. Wiley: Brunner/Mazel, 1982.

Ginneken, Jaap van. *Crowds, Psychology, and Politics: 1871–1899.* Cambridge: Cambridge UP, 1992.

Goodrich, B. F. *A Wonder Book of Rubber.* Akron: Superior Printing, 1917.

Gould, George M., and Walter L. Pyle. *Anomalies and Curiosities of Medicine.* Philadelphia: Saunders, 1901.

"The Gratuitous Exhibitions of London: No. II." *Punch* 3–4 (1842–43): 194–95.

"The Gratuitous Exhibitions of London: Preliminary." *Punch* 3–4 (1842–43): 179–80.

Gray, Chris Hables, ed. *The Cyborg Handbook.* New York: Routledge, 1995.

Gray, Chris Hables, and Steven Mentor. "The Cyborg Body Politic and the New World Order." In Brahm and Driscoll, eds., *Prosthetic Territories*, 219–47.

"The Great American Humbug." *Tait's Edinburgh Magazine* (February 1855): 73–81.

Greenblatt, Stephen. *Learning to Curse: Essays in Early Modern Culture.* New York: Routledge, 1990.

Greenhow, E. H. *Papers Relating to the Sanitary State of the People of England, General Board of Health, London 1858.* Farnborough, Hants.: Gregg International, 1973.

Greg, W. R. "Prostitution." *Westminster Review* 53 (1850): 448–506.

Gross, Samuel. *A Practical Treatise on Tumors of the Mammary Gland: Embracing Their Histology, Pathology, Diagnosis, and Treatment.* New York: Appleton, 1880.

Grossberg, Lawrence. "Toward a Genealogy of the State of Cultural Studies: The Discipline of Communication and the Reception of Cultural Studies in the United States." In *Disciplinarity and Dissent in Cultural Studies,* ed. Cary Nelson and Dilip Parameshwar Gaonkar, 131–47. New York: Routledge, 1996.

—. *We Gotta Get out of This Place: Popular Conservatism and Postmodern Culture.* New York: Routledge, 1992.

Grossberg, Lawrence, Cary Nelson, and Paula A. Treichler, eds. *Cultural Studies.* New York: Routledge, 1992.

Grosz, Elisabeth. "Intolerable Ambiguity: Freaks as/at the Limit." In Thomson, ed., *Freakery,* 55–66.

Grove, William Robert. *The Correlation of Physical Forces.* 6th ed. London: Longmans, Green, 1874.

Guillory, John. "Preprofessionalism: What Graduate Students Want." *Profession 1996,* 91–99.

Haley, Bruce. *The Healthy Body and Victorian Culture.* Cambridge: Harvard UP, 1978.

Halttunen, Karen. *Confidence Men and Painted Women: A Study of Middle-Class Culture in America, 1830–1870.* New Haven: Yale UP, 1982.

Hamlin, Christopher. *A Science of Impurity: Water Analysis in Nineteenth-Century Britain.* Berkeley: U California P, 1990.

Haraway, Donna. "The Promises of Monsters: A Regenerative Politics for Inappropriate/d Others." In Grossberg, Nelson, and Treichler, eds., *Cultural Studies,* 295–337.

Harris, Neil. *Humbug: The Art of P. T. Barnum.* Boston: Little, Brown, 1973.

Hemyng, Bracebridge. "Prostitution in London." In Mayhew, *London Labour and the London Poor,* 4:210–72.

Hobsbawm, Eric. *Industry and Empire:*

The Making of Modern English Society: 1750 to the Present Day. New York: Pantheon, 1968.

Hollingshead, John. "People's Umbrellas [as indices to character]." *Household Words* 17 (1858): 496–98.

Hone, William. *The Every-day Book and Table Book, or Everlasting Calendar of Popular Amusements, Sports, Pastimes, Ceremonies, Manners, Customs, and Events*. Vol. 1. London: Griffin, 1837–38.

Huet, Marie-Hélène. *Monstrous Imagination*. Cambridge: Harvard UP, 1993.

Huggins, G. Martin. *Amputation Stumps: Their Care and After-Treatment*. London: Henry Frowde, Hodder and Stoughton, 1918.

Hunter, Dianne. "Hysteria, Psychoanalysis, and Feminism: The Case of Anna O." In *The (M)other Tongue: Essays in Feminist Psychoanalytic Interpretation*, ed. Shirley Nelson Garner, Claire Kahane, and Madelon Sprengnether, 89–115. Ithaca: Cornell UP, 1985.

Hutcheon, Linda. "Circling the Downspout of Empire: Post-colonialism and Postmodernism." *Ariel* 20 (1989): 149–75.

Hutter, Albert D. "Dismemberment and Articulation in *Our Mutual Friend*." *Dickens Studies Annual: Essays on Victorian Fiction* 11 (1983): 135–75.

"Improved Artificial Limbs." *Scientific American* 72 (1895): 52. (Reprinted in Marks, *Treatise on Artificial Limbs*, 360.)

Jackson, James Jr. *Cases of Cholera Collected at Paris, in the Month of April 1832, in the Wards of MM. Andral and Louis, at the Hospital La Pitié*. Boston: Carter, Hendee, 1832.

Jacobus, Mary. "Baring the Breast: Mastectomy and the Surgical Analogy." In *First Things: The Maternal Imaginary in Literature, Art, and Psychoanalysis*, 231–67. New York: Routledge, 1995.

Jacobus, Mary, Evelyn Fox Keller, and Sally Shuttleworth, eds. *Body/Politics: Women and the Discourses of Science*. New York: Routledge, 1990.

James, William. "The Consciousness of Lost Limbs." In *Essays in Psychology*, 204–15. Cambridge: Harvard UP, 1983.

Jameson, Horatio Gates. *Treatise on Epidemic Cholera*. Philadelphia: Lindsay and Blakiston, 1855.

Jerrold, William Blanchard. "The Iron Seamstress." *Household Words* 8 (1854): 575–76.

Johnson, Barbara. "My Monster/My Self." *Diacritics* 12 (1982): 2–10.

Johnson, Sir George. *Notes on Cholera: Its Nature and Its Treatment*. London: Longmans, Green, 1866.

Johnson, Richard. "What Is Cultural Studies Anyway?" *Social Text* 16 (1987): 38–80.

Jordanova, Ludmilla. *Sexual Visions: Images of Gender in Science and Medicine between the Eighteenth and Twentieth Centuries*. Madison: U Wisconsin P, 1989.

Katz, Leslie. "Flesh of His Flesh: Amputation in *Moby Dick* and S. W. Mitchell's Medical Papers." *Genders* 4 (spring 1989): 1–10.

Kay, James Phillips. *The Moral and Physical Condition of the Working Classes Employed in the Cotton Manufacture in Manchester*. 1832. 2d ed. London: Frank Cass, 1970.

Keating, Peter, ed. *Into Unknown England 1866–1913: Selections from the Social Explorers*. Manchester: Manchester UP, 1976.

Keller, Evelyn Fox, and Helen E. Lon-

gino, eds. *Feminism & Science.* Oxford:
Oxford UP, 1996.

Kent, Christopher. "Victorian Social History: Post-Thompson, Post-Foucault,
Postmodern." *Victorian Studies* 40 (autumn 1996): 97–133.

Ketabgian, Tamara. "The Human Pros-
thesis: Workers and Machines in the
Victorian Industrial Scene." *Critical
Matrix* 11 (1997): 4–32.

Kingsley, Charles. *Charles Kingsley, His
Letters and Memories of His Life.* 1877.
Vol. 2. New York: AMS, 1973.

—. "Cheap Clothes and Nasty." Reprinted
in Kingsley, *Alton Locke: Tailor and Poet.*
New York: Harper, 1850.

—. *The Water Babies.* 1863. Harmondsworth: Penguin, 1984.

—. "The Water Supply of London."
North British Review 25, no. 29 (1851):
117–30.

Koven, Seth. "Remembering and Dismemberment: Crippled Children,
Wounded Soldiers, and the Great War
in Great Britain." *American Historical
Review* (October 1994): 1167–1202.

Kucich, John. *Repression in Victorian Fic-
tion: Charlotte Brontë, George Eliot, and
Charles Dickens.* Berkeley: U California
P, 1987.

Kumar, Anil. *Medicine and the Raj: British
Medical Policy in India, 1835–1911.* New
Delhi: Sage, 1998.

Kunhardt, Philip. *P. T. Barnum: America's
Greatest Showman.* New York: Knopf,
1995.

Laqueur, Thomas. *Making Sex: Body and
Gender from the Greeks to Freud.* Cambridge: Harvard UP, 1990.

Le Bon, Gustave. *The Crowd: A Study of
the Popular Mind.* 2d ed. Dunwoody,
GA: Norman S. Berg, 1968. (Originally

published as *Psychologie des foules*
[1895].)

Leech, John. "A Court for King Cholera."
Punch 23 (1852): 139.

Levy, Anita. *Other Women: The Writing of
Class, Race, and Gender, 1832–1898.*
Princeton: Princeton UP, 1991.

Lewes, George Henry. *Problems of Life and
Mind.* 3d ser. Boston: Houghton, Os-
good, 1879–80.

Lindfors, Bernth. "Ethnological Show
Business: Footlighting the Dark Continent." In Thomson, ed., *Freakery,*
207–18.

Lombroso, Cesare. *L'uomo delinquente.*
1876. Rome: Napoleone, 1971.

Longmate, Norman. *King Cholera: The
Biography of a Disease.* London: Hamish
Hamilton, 1966.

Lynn, Eliza. "Why Is the Negro Black?"
Household Words 15 (1857): 587–88.

McClintock, Anne. *Imperial Leather: Race,
Gender, and Sexuality in the Colonial
Contest.* New York: Routledge, 1995.

"M. Culloch and MacLaren on Cholera."
Littell's Living Age 27 (1850): 24–25.

McKim, W. Duncan. *Heredity and Human
Progress.* New York: Putnam, 1900.

McLaughlin, Terence. *Coprophilia; or, A
Peck of Dirt.* London: Cassell, 1971.

MacLeod, Roy M., and Milton James
Lewis, eds. *Disease, Medicine and Empire: Perspectives on Western Medicine
and the Experience of European Expansion.* London: Routledge, 1988.

McNeill, William H. *Plagues and Peoples.*
New York: Doubleday, 1977.

Mangan, J. A., and James Walvin, eds.
*Manliness and Morality: Middle-Class
Masculinity in Britain and America,
1800–1940.* New York: St. Martin's,
1987.

Mann, Thomas. *Death in Venice and Seven Other Stories*. Trans. H. T. Lowe-Porter. New York: Random House, Vintage Books, 1936.

Mansfield, Carl M. *Early Breast Cancer: Its History and Results of Treatment*. Basel, NY: Karger, 1976.

"The Manufacture of Artificial Limbs." *Scientific American* (1895). (Reprinted in Marks, *Treatise on Artificial Limbs*, 360–68.)

Marks, A. A. *A Treatise on Artificial Limbs with Rubber Hands and Feet*. New York: A. A. Marks, 1903.

—. *A Treatise on Marks' Patent Artificial Limbs with Rubber Hands and Feet*. New York: A. A. Marks, 1888.

Martin, Emily. "The Egg and the Sperm: How Science Has Constructed a Romance Based on Stereotypical Male-Female Roles." In Keller and Longino, eds. *Feminism & Science*, 103–17.

Marx, Karl. *Capital: A Critique of Political Economy*. 1867. Trans. Ben Fowkes. Harmondsworth: Penguin, 1976.

—. *The Eighteenth Brumaire of Louis Bonaparte*. In *Marx-Engels Selected Works*, vol. 1. London: Lawrence and Wishart, 1951.

Masterman, C. F. G. *The Condition of England*. 3d ed. London: Methuen, 1909.

Maudsley, Henry. *Body and Mind*. New York: D. Appleton, 1871.

Mayhew, Henry. *London Labour and the London Poor*. 1861. 4 vols. London: Griffin, Bohn, 1861.

—. "A Visit to the Cholera Districts of Bermondsey." In *The Morning Chronicle Survey of Labour and the Poor: The Metropolitan Districts*, 1:31–39. East Sussex: Redwood Burn, 1980.

Meredith, George. *The Egoist*. 1879. New York: New American Library, 1963.

—. *The Ordeal of Richard Feverel*. 1859. New York: Dover, 1983.

Michaels, Walter Benn. *The Gold Standard and the Logic of Naturalism: American Literature at the Turn of the Century*. Berkeley: U California P, 1987.

Miklitsch, Robert. Letter. Forum on Cultural Studies and the Literary. *PMLA* 112 (March 1997): 257–58.

Miller, D. A. "The Late Jane Austen." *Raritan* 10 (summer 1990): 55–79.

—. *The Novel and the Police*. Berkeley: U California P, 1988.

Millett, Kate. *Sexual Politics*. Garden City, NY: Doubleday, 1970.

Mitchell, Silas Weir. *The Autobiography of a Quack and Other Stories*. New York: Century, 1905.

—. "The Case of George Dedlow." *Atlantic Monthly* 18 (1866): 1–11.

—. *Injuries of Nerves and Their Consequences*. 1872. New York: Dover, 1965.

—. *Lectures on Diseases of the Nervous System, Especially in Women*. Philadelphia: Lea, 1885.

—. "Phantom Limbs." *Lippincott's Magazine of Popular Literature and Science* 8 (1871): 563–69.

Moers, Ellen. *Literary Women*. Garden City, NY: Doubleday, 1976.

"More Dwarfs." *Punch* 10 (1846): 93.

Morris, David B. *The Culture of Pain*. Berkeley: U California P, 1991.

Morris, R. J. *Cholera, 1832: A Social Response to an Epidemic*. London: Croom Helm, 1976.

Mort, Frank. *Dangerous Sexualities: Medico-Moral Politics in England since 1830*. London: Routledge and Kegan Paul, 1987.

Moulin, Daniel de. *A Short History of Breast Cancer*. Boston: Nijhoff, 1983.

"Mr. Simon's Report—Nature of the Cholera Poison." *Littell's Living Age* 40 (1854): 428–31.

Mullan, John. *Sentiment and Sociability: The Language of Feeling in the Eighteenth Century.* Oxford: Clarendon, 1988.

Nelson, Robert. *Asiatic Cholera: Its Origin and Spread in Asia, Africa, and Europe, Introduced into America through Canada; Remote and Proximate Causes, Symptoms and Pathology, and the Various Modes of Treatment Analyzed.* New York: William A. Townsend, 1866.

Newton, Robert. Introduction to Shapter, *The History of the Cholera in Exeter in 1832.*

Nunn, Thomas William. *On Cancer of the Breast.* London: Churchill, 1882.

Nye, Robert A. *The Origins of Crowd Psychology: Gustave Le Bon and the Crisis of Mass Democracy in the Third Republic.* London: Sage, 1975.

Official Descriptive and Illustrated Catalogue of the Great Exhibition of the Works of Industry of All Nations, 1851. London: Spicer Brothers, 1851.

"On the Disadvantages of Not Being a Dwarf." *Douglas Jerrold's Shilling Magazine* (1846): 326–30.

Oppenheim, Janet. *The Other World: Spiritualism and Psychical Research in England, 1850–1914.* Cambridge: Cambridge UP, 1985.

—. *"Shattered Nerves": Doctors, Patients, and Depression in Victorian England.* New York: Oxford UP, 1991.

Oppenheimer, Jane M. "Some Historical Relationships between Teratology and Experimental Embryology." *Bulletin of the History of Medicine* 42 (1968): 145–59.

Orbach, Susie. *Hunger Strike: The Anorectic's Struggle as a Metaphor for Our Age.* New York: Norton, 1986.

Otis, Laura. *Membranes: Metaphors of Invasion in Nineteenth-Century Literature, Science, and Politics.* Baltimore: Johns Hopkins UP, 1999.

Owen, Alex. *The Darkened Room: Women, Power, and Spiritualism in Late Victorian England.* Philadelphia: U Pennsylvania P, 1990.

Paget, James. *Clinical Lectures and Essays.* London: Longmans, Green, 1875.

—. *Lectures on Surgical Pathology.* 1865. 3d American ed. Philadelphia: Lindsay and Blakiston, 1876.

Parker, Willard. *Cancer: A Study of Three Hundred and Ninety-seven Cases of Cancer of the Female Breast.* New York: Putnam, 1885.

Pearson, Karl. *The Life, Letters and Labours of Francis Galton.* 2 vols. Cambridge: Cambridge UP, 1924.

Pelling, Margaret. *Cholera, Fever and English Medicine, 1825–1865.* Oxford: Oxford UP, 1978.

Pernick, Martin. "Back from the Grave: Recurring Controversies over Defining and Diagnosing Death in History." In *Death: Beyond Whole-Brain Criteria,* ed. Richard Zaner, 17–74. Kluwer, 1988.

Perry, Ruth. *The Celebrated Mary Astell: An Early English Feminist.* Chicago: U Chicago P, 1986.

—. "Colonizing the Breast: Sexuality and Maternity in Eighteenth-Century England." *Eighteenth-Century Life* 16 (February 1992): 185–213.

Peters, John C. *Notes on the Origin, Nature, Prevention, and Treatment of Asiatic Cholera.* 2d ed. New York: D. Van Nostrand, 1867.

Pick, Daniel. *Faces of Degeneration: A European Disorder, c. 1848–1918*. New York: Cambridge UP, 1989.

Poe, Edgar Allan. "The Man That Was Used Up." In *The Complete Works of Edgar Allan Poe*, 3:259–72. New York: Kelmscott Society, 1902.

Poovey, Mary. *Making a Social Body: British Cultural Formation, 1830–1864*. Chicago: U Chicago P, 1995.

—. "Scenes of an Indelicate Character: The Medical Treatment of Victorian Women." In Poovey, *Uneven Developments*, 24–50.

—. *Uneven Developments: The Ideological Work of Gender in Mid-Victorian England*. Chicago: U Chicago P, 1988.

Porter, Carolyn. "Are We Being Historical Yet?" *SAQ* 87 (fall 1988): 743–86.

—. "History and Literature: 'After the New Historicism.'" *New Literary History* 21 (winter 1990): 253–72.

Power, D'Arcy. "The History of the Amputation of the Breast to 1904." *Liverpool Medico-Chirurgical Journal* 42 (1934): 29–56.

Price, Douglas B. "Miraculous Restoration of Lost Body Parts: Relationship to the Phantom Limb Phenomenon and to Limb-Burial Superstitions and Practices." In *American Folk Medicine: A Symposium*, ed. Wayland D. Hand, 49–71. Berkeley: U California P, 1976.

Price, Douglas B., and Neil J. Twombly, eds. *The Phantom Limb Phenomenon: A Medical, Folkloric, and Historical Study*. Washington, D.C.: Georgetown UP, 1978.

Rabinbach, Anson. *The Human Motor: Energy, Fatigue, and the Origins of Modernity*. Berkeley: U California P, 1992.

Rather, L. J., ed. *Disease, Life, and Man: Selected Essays by Rudolf Virchow*. Stanford: Stanford UP, 1958.

—. *The Genesis of Cancer: A Study in the History of Ideas*. Baltimore: Johns Hopkins UP, 1978.

—. "Harvey, Virchow, Bernard, and the Methodology of Science." In Rather, *Disease, Life, and Man*. 1–25.

—. "The Place of Virchow's 'Cellular Pathology' in Medical Thought." In Virchow, *Cellular Pathology*, v–xxvii.

Reid, Donald. *Paris Sewers and Sewermen: Realities and Representations*. Cambridge: Harvard UP, 1991.

"Report on the Sanitary Conditions of the Labouring Classes." *Quarterly Review* 71 (1842): 417–53.

"Revelations of a Showman." *Blackwood's Edinburgh Magazine* 77 (1855): 187–201.

Richards, Evelleen. "A Political Anatomy of Monsters, Hopeful and Otherwise: Teratogeny, Transcendentalism, and Evolutionary Theorizing." *Isis* 85 (1994): 377–411.

Richards, Thomas. *The Commodity Culture of Victorian England: Advertising and Spectacle, 1851–1914*. Stanford: Stanford UP, 1990.

Richardson, Ruth. *Death, Dissection and the Destitute*. Harmondsworth: Penguin, 1988.

Rideing, William H. "Patched-up Humanity." *Appleton's Journal* 13 (1875): 783–84. (Reprinted in Marks, *Treatise on Marks' Patent Artificial Limbs*, 150–52.)

Riis, Jacob. *How the Other Half Lives: Studies among the Tenements of New York*. 1890. Cambridge: Belknap, 1970.

Robbins, Bruce. *Secular Vocations: Intellectuals, Professionalism, Culture*. London: Verso, 1993.

Robbins, Guy, ed. *Silvergirl's Surgery: The Breast.* Austin, TX: Silvergirl, 1984.

Rogers, Blair O. "Carl Ferdinand von Graefe." *Journal of Plastic and Reconstructive Surgery* 46 (1970): 554–63.

Ronell, Avital. *The Telephone Book: Technology, Schizophrenia, Electric Speech.* Lincoln: U Nebraska P, 1989.

Rosenberg, Charles E. *The Cholera Years: The United States in 1832, 1849, and 1866.* Chicago: U Chicago P, 1987.

—. *Explaining Epidemics and Other Studies in the History of Medicine.* Cambridge: Cambridge UP, 1992.

Rowley, J. F. *An Illustrated Treatise on Artificial Legs with Patent Wax Sockets.* Chicago, 1911.

Ruskin, John. *"Unto this Last": Four Essays on the First Principles of Political Economy.* New York: John Wiley and Son, 1866.

Russett, Cynthia Eagle. *Sexual Science: The Victorian Construction of Womanhood.* Cambridge: Harvard UP, 1989.

Russo, Mary. *The Female Grotesque: Risk, Excess, and Modernity.* New York: Routledge, 1995.

Said, Edward W. *Culture and Imperialism.* New York: Knopf, 1993.

—. *Orientalism.* New York: Pantheon, 1978.

—. *The World, the Text, and the Critic.* Cambridge: Harvard UP, 1983.

Saint-Hilaire, Geoffroy. *Histoire générale et particulière des anomalies de l'organisation chez l'homme et les animaux.* Paris: J.-B. Baillière, 1832.

Saint-Hilaire, Geoffroy, and Georges Cuvier. *Histoire naturelle des mammifères avec des figures originales.* Paris: Belin, 1924.

"Sanitary Consolidation." *Quarterly Review* 88 (1850): 435–92.

"Sanitary Reform." *Edinburgh Review* 91 (1849): 210–28.

Saxon, A. H. *P. T. Barnum: The Legend and the Man.* New York: Columbia UP, 1989.

Scarry, Elaine. *The Body in Pain: The Making and Unmaking of the World.* New York: Oxford UP, 1985.

Schiebinger, Londa. *Nature's Body: Gender in the Making of Modern Science.* Boston: Beacon, 1993.

Schudson, Michael. "Paper Tigers." *Lingua Franca* 7 (August 1997): 49–56.

Scott, Joan Wallach. *Gender and the Politics of History.* New York: Columbia UP, 1988.

Sedgwick, Eve Kosofsky. *Epistemology of the Closet.* Berkeley: U California P, 1990.

Seltzer, Mark. *Bodies and Machines.* New York: Routledge, 1992.

—. "Serial Killers (1)." *differences: A Journal of Feminist Cultural Studies* 5, no. 1 (1993): 92–128.

Shapter, Thomas. *The History of the Cholera in Exeter in 1832.* 1849. Wakefield: S.R. Publishers, 1971.

Sheild, Arthur Marmaduke. *A Clinical Treatise on Diseases of the Breast.* London: Macmillan, 1898.

Shorter, Edward. *From Paralysis to Fatigue: A History of Psychosomatic Illness in the Modern Era.* New York: Free Press, 1992.

Showalter, Elaine. *The Female Malady: Women, Madness, and Culture in England, 1830–1980.* New York: Pantheon, 1985.

—. *A Literature of Their Own: British Women Novelists from Brontë to Lessing.* Princeton: Princeton UP, 1976.

Shuttleworth, Sally. "Female Circulation: Medical Discourse and Popular Advertising in the Mid-Victorian Era." In Jacobus, Keller, and Shuttleworth, eds., *Body/Politics*, 47–68.

Siegfried, J., and M. Zimmermann, eds. *Phantom and Stump Pain.* New York: Springer-Verlag, 1981.

Simpson, David, ed. *Subject to History: Ideology, Class, Gender.* Ithaca: Cornell UP, 1991.

Sloane, T. O'Conor. *Rubber Hand Stamps and the Manipulation of India Rubber.* New York: Henley, 1890.

Smith, Thomas Southwood. *Treatise on Fever.* Philadelphia: Carey and Lea, 1830.

Smith, William. *Advertise: How? When? Where?* London: Routledge, Warne, and Routledge, 1863.

Smith-Rosenberg, Carroll. *Disorderly Conduct: Visions of Gender in Victorian America.* New York: Oxford UP, 1985.

Snow, John. *On the Mode of Communication of Cholera.* 2nd ed., much enlarged. London: Churchill, 1855.

Sontag, Susan. *Illness as Metaphor; and AIDS and Its Metaphors.* New York: Anchor, 1989.

"Spasmodic Cholera." *Westminster Review* 15 (1831): 484–90.

Stallybrass, Peter, and Allon White. *The Politics and Poetics of Transgression.* Ithaca: Cornell UP, 1986.

Steedman, Carolyn. "Culture, Cultural Studies, and the Historians." In Grossberg, Nelson, and Treichler, eds., *Cultural Studies*, 613–22.

—. *Strange Dislocations: Childhood and the Idea of Human Interiority, 1780–1930.* Cambridge: Harvard UP, 1995.

Stepan, Nancy Leys. "Race and Gender: The Role of Analogy in Science." In Keller and Longino, eds., *Feminism & Science*, 121–36.

Stevenson, Robert Louis. *Dr. Jekyll and Mr. Hyde.* 1885. Harmondsworth: Penguin, 1979.

—. "The Philosophy of Umbrellas." Reprinted in *Essays Literary and Critical.* London: W. Heinemann, 1925.

Stewart, Susan. *On Longing: Narratives of the Miniature, the Gigantic, the Souvenir, the Collection.* Durham: Duke UP, 1993.

Stocking, George W. Jr. *Victorian Anthropology.* New York: Free Press, 1987.

Stone, Sandy. "Split Subjects, Not Atoms; or, How I Fell in Love with My Prosthesis." In Gray, ed., *The Cyborg Handbook*, 393–406.

"Supply of Water to the Metropolis." *Edinburgh Review* 91 (1849): 377–408.

Sweeting, Richard. "On a New Operation for Cancer of the Breast." *Lancet* 1 (1869): 323. (Reprinted in Robbins, ed., *Silvergirl's Surgery: The Breast, 78.)

Talbot, Eugene S. *Degeneracy: Its Causes, Signs, and Results, 1898.* New York: Garland, 1984.

Tardieu, Ambroise. *Treatise on Epidemic Cholera.* Trans. Samuel Lee Bigelow. Boston: Ticknor, Reed and Fields, 1849.

Tarnowsky, Pauline. *Étude anthropométrique sur les prostituées et les voleuses.* Paris: Progrès Medical, 1889.

Thackeray, William Makepeace. *The History of Henry Esmond, Esq.* 1852. London: Smith, Elder, 1868.

Thackrah, Charles Turner. *The Effects of Arts, Trades, and Professions on Health and Longevity.* 1832. Canton, MA: Science History Publications, 1985.

Thompson, E. P. *The Making of the English Working Class.* New York: Knopf, 1966.

Thomson, Rosemarie Garland. *Extraordinary Bodies: Figuring Physical Disability in American Culture and Literature*. New York: Columbia UP, 1997.

—, ed. *Freakery: Cultural Spectacles of the Extraordinary Body*. New York: New York UP, 1996.

Todd, Dennis. *Imagining Monsters: Miscreations of the Self in Eighteenth-Century England*. Chicago: U Chicago P, 1995.

Trollope, Anthony. *He Knew He Was Right*. 1869. Oxford: Oxford UP, 1992.

Twain, Mark. "Personal Habits of the Siamese Twins." In *Sketches New and Old*. Hartford: American Publishing Co., 1875.

—. *Pudd'nhead Wilson and Those Extraordinary Twins*. 1894. Harmondsworth: Penguin, 1987.

Twitchell, James. *Carnival Culture: The Trashing of Taste in America*. New York: Columbia UP, 1992.

"Umbrellas." *Gentleman's Magazine* (June 1889): 536–44.

"Umbrellas in the East." *Penny Magazine* (December 1835): 479–80.

Ure, Andrew. *The Philosophy of Manufactures; or, An Exposition of the Scientific, Moral, and Commercial Economy of the Factory System of Great Britain*. 1835. London: Frank Cass, 1967.

Veith, Ilza. *Hysteria: The History of a Disease*. Chicago: U Chicago P, 1965.

Velpeau, Alfred Armand Louis Marie. *A Treatise on the Diseases of the Breast*. Trans. S. Parkman. Philadelphia: Waldie, 1840.

Vicinus, Martha, ed. *Suffer and Be Still: Women in the Victorian Age*. Bloomington: Indiana UP, 1972.

—, ed. *A Widening Sphere: Changing Roles of Victorian Women*. Bloomington: Indiana UP, 1977.

Virchow, Rudolf. "Atoms and Individuals" (1859). In Rather, ed., *Disease, Life, and Man*, 120–41.

—. "Cellular Pathology" (1855). In Rather, ed., *Disease, Life, and Man*, 71–101.

—. *Cellular Pathology as Based upon Physiological and Pathological Histology*. Trans. Frank Chance. New York: Dover, 1971.

—. "On the Mechanistic Interpretation of Life" (1858). In Rather, ed., *Disease, Life, and Man*, 102–19.

Vrettos, Athena. *Somatic Fictions: Imagining Illness in Victorian Culture*. Stanford: Stanford UP, 1995.

Walkowitz, Judith. *Prostitution and Victorian Society: Women, Class, and the State*. Cambridge: Cambridge UP, 1980.

Ward, Edward T. "Gamps." *Dickensian* 24 (winter 1927–28): 41–43.

Warren, Samuel. "Passages from the Diary of a Late Physician: A Cancer." *Blackwood's Edinburgh Magazine* 18 (September 1830): 474–76.

Watson, B. A. *A Treatise on Amputations of the Extremities and Their Complications*. Philadelphia: P. Blakiston, 1885.

Weeks, Jeffrey. *Sex, Politics, and Society: The Regulation of Sexuality since 1800*. New York: Longman, 1989.

Wendt, Edmund Charles. *A Treatise on Asiatic Cholera*. New York: William Wood, 1885.

Wigley, Mark. "Prosthetic Theory: The Disciplining of Architecture." *Assemblage* 15 (1991): 7–29.

Wills, David. *Prosthesis*. Stanford: Stanford UP, 1995.

Wohl, Anthony S. *Endangered Lives: Public Health in Victorian Britain*. Cambridge: Harvard UP, 1983.

Wolf, Naomi. *The Beauty Myth: How Images of Beauty Are Used against Women.* New York: Morrow, 1991.

Wood, E. J. *Giants and Dwarfs.* London: Richard Bentley, 1868.

Woodruff, William. *The Rise of the British Rubber Industry during the Nineteenth Century.* Liverpool: Liverpool UP, 1958.

Wordsworth, William. *The Prelude.* 1850. New York: Norton, 1979.

Yalom, Marilyn. *A History of the Breast.* New York: Knopf, 1997.

Erin O'Connor is Assistant Professor of English
at the University of Pennsylvania.

Library of Congress Cataloging-in-Publication Data
O'Connor, Erin, 1968–
    Raw material : producing pathology in Victorian culture /
Erin O'Connor.
        p. cm. — (Body, commodity, text)
    Includes bibliographical references and index.
    ISBN 0-8223-2608-6 (cloth : alk. paper)
    ISBN 0-8223-2616-7 (pbk. : alk. paper)
    1. Social medicine—England—History—19th century.
    2. Medicine, Industrial—England—History—19th century.
    3. Cholera—England—History—19th century.
    4. Communicable diseases—Social aspects—England—
History—19th century.
    5. Public health—Social aspects—England—History—
19th century.
    I. Title. II. Series.
RA418.3.G7 O26 2001
610'.942'09034—dc21
00-030308